The Longevity Factor

CHROMIUM PICOLINATE

Other Recent Books by Dr. Passwater

Chromium Picolinate (a Good Health Guide)

Cancer Prevention and Nutritional Therapies
The New Superantioxidant — Plus
(a Good Health Guide)

The New Supernutrition

The Longevity Factor
CHROMIUM PICOLINATE

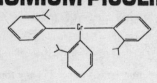

Richard A. Passwater, Ph.D.

Keats Publishing, Inc.　　　New Canaan, Connecticut

The Longevity Factor is not intended as medical advice. Its intent is solely informational and educational. Please consult a health professional should the need for one be indicated.

THE LONGEVITY FACTOR

Library of Congress Cataloging-in-Publication Data
Passwater, Richard A.
    The longevity factor: chromium picolinate/Richard A Passwater.
        p.   cm.
    Cover title: Living longer, living better, slowing aging with the longevity factor.
    Includes bibliographical references and index.
    ISBN 0-87983-619-9 $4.95
    1. Chromium in human nutrition.   2. Chromium – Physiological effect.   3. Longevity.   I. Title   II. Title: Living longer, living better, slowing aging with the longevity factor.
QP535.C7P38   1993   93-5147
612.6'8 – dc20   CIP

Printed in the United States of America

Published by Keats Publishing, Inc.
27 Pine Street (Box 876)
New Canaan, Connecticut 06840-0876

CONTENTS

1

The Chromium Picolinate Promise

*It is often necessary to make decisions on the basis
of information sufficient for action, but insufficient to
satisfy the intellect.*

Immanuel Kant

TIMING is everything. Even with knowledge, timing is
critical. We can wait a hundred years to find out for sure,
but will it do us any good? There have been several very
interesting scientific discoveries that promise to have a
major impact on how long we live and how well we live.
The purpose of this book is to tell you about these discoveries, so that you may make a very important decision —
now, while there is still time for *you* to benefit.

Spectacular evidence is rapidly accumulating that an
especially bioactive form of a specific nutrient can help optimize your body chemistry, enabling you to live longer, with
less risk of age-associated diseases, with more vigor, and
even with a more youthful-appearing physique. The critical
nutrient is the mineral chromium, and the form proven to be
so biologically effective is chromium picolinate.

Studies show chromium picolinate dramatically
increases the lifespan of animals. In human clinical studies,
it lowers heart disease risk, helps burn away excess body
fat, increases muscularity, and produces many other beneficial effects. All of these benefits are without risk;
chromium picolinate is one of the safest nutrients ever
tested and only tiny (microgram) amounts are needed.

This is not an arcane scientific treatise. It is a plain
explanation of the important facts so that you may under-

stand the research and the scientific basis of my enthusiasm. The confirming studies and further refinement of the theory are under way. This is merely a communication to those interested in better health and a longer, fuller life, at a time early enough to benefit them.

I wish that I could report to you that chromium picolinate has already been shown to increase the lifespan of humans, but by the time we agree on an ethical way to conduct the study, and then follow groups of middle-aged persons — some taking chromium picolinate and others not — throughout the remainder of their lives, many decades will have passed.

No matter how many animal studies we conduct, scientists will always say they may not be relevant to humans, because we are not rodents, guinea pigs or dogs. It won't be *proven* unequivocally until we conduct century-long longevity studies with chromium picolinate in actual humans.

This is the problem that I ran into with my gerontological studies in the late 1960s. I had consistently shown that synergistic amounts of specific antioxidant nutrients increased the average lifespan of rodents. My colleagues told me that this information probably wouldn't apply to man. I was told that I should conduct studies on various species, including primates, using any success from one species as a basis to get a grant for a similar study in the next-closest species.

Well, this is how scientists keep funded and promoted as they become the experts in a line of study. However, most studies are conducted over months, not decades. I realized that even when I showed monkeys living far longer, I would still have to prove that it would work with people.

Not having nine lives or nine million dollars, I decided that if I were ever going to help anybody, I would have to make some prudent decisions based on less than ultimate scientific evidence. In Toronto, on October 23, 1970, at the

Gerontological Society's 23rd Annual Meeting, I presented an alternative way to measure the aging process in man, which shortened the study time to merely one decade.[1] But alas, even then the funding institutions did not think that such a study was a good investment.

Shortly, I will explain why slowing the aging process is your very best health investment. Slowing aging also means that the age-associated diseases can be prevented. We get older without getting old. It means that we can be more productive longer. We are younger longer. It is not just more years in our lives, it is more life in our years. It greatly reduces the expenses of old age. Slowing the aging process means extending the good years of healthy middle age and greatly decreasing the bad years of old age. I'll explain how this works later.

Now there are many scientists who believe, and massive evidence indicates, that the antioxidant nutrients such as the trace mineral selenium and vitamins A, C, and E protect against heart disease and cancer, and indeed, help us live longer. Government agencies are now funding the first human clinical studies to confirm that antioxidant nutrients do indeed protect real people from cancer and heart disease. In a few decades, we should have confirming data.

Oh, you say you know about how antioxidant nutrients protect against heart disease and cancer? Well, the final proof isn't in yet. Oh, you say you have seen enough good evidence to make the prudent judgment to supplement your diet with antioxidants — just like the scientists who research this field? OK — but this is the mid-nineties. It's a shame that you didn't start 20 years sooner. You could have, if you had followed my research findings.

In 1970, I taught how to prevent age-associated damage by reducing the harm caused by free radicals. This advice was based on my own research and the research of Drs. Denham Harman, Al Tappel and two or three other researchers. As you probably know, this research has now been confirmed in thousands of studies by hundreds of researchers. One major process that accelerates aging occurs when oxygen radicals cause a change in body proteins to produce "*oxygen*-damaged" proteins. To lessen damage from free radicals, you merely need to optimize your antioxidant nutrient intake. This approach has proved to be very effective against secondary aging effects, and can lead to an additional 5 to 15 years of disease prevention and life.

I am teaching how to prevent age-associated damage by reducing the harm caused by fluctuations in blood sugar to produce what are called "*sugar*-damaged" proteins. This advice is based on the research of others and has been confirmed by dozens of studies. To lessen damage from sugar-damaged proteins, one merely needs to optimize chromium intake with chromium picolinate. Alternately, one can choose to severely restrict caloric intake to fewer than 1,500 calories per day. I don't advocate severe calorie restriction, which requires an iron will, but I do recommend supplemental antioxidant nutrients. The chromium picolinate approach by itself promises better results than either calorie restriction or antioxidants individually. Evidence also suggests that the chromium picolinate and antioxidant approaches may be used together with synergistic results.

The chromium picolinate approach is the superior approach because it not only modifies the secondary aging effects, it very probably slows the primary aging process. This regimen may well exceed a 10- to 15-year increase in longevity. Only time will tell.

In my laboratory animal studies with antioxidant nutrients, I could produce significant (30 percent) increases in *average* lifespans of animals fed a diet high in antioxidants compared to the controls fed the same diet with normal amounts of antioxidants, but only meager (5-10 percent) increases in maximum lifespan.[2] In the experiments where the control animals lived normal lifespans, the improvements were not as great. This indicated that the antioxidants were not slowing the fundamental aging process, but were protecting the animals against environmental effects that shorten life. As I later determined, the increases in average lifespans were primarily due to protection against cancer, liver damage, pollutants, and other stresses.

However, with chromium picolinate there has been a dramatic 36 percent increase in average lifespan and a 17 percent increase (over controls) in maximum lifespan. This is direct evidence of slowing the aging process itself.

Remember, it is not simply living longer. Both approaches reduce the incidence of the "aging diseases," including heart disease. They are complementary approaches that enhance each other's benefits. As an example, antioxidants are very effective in preventing cancer, and chromium picolinate is very effective in preventing the damage caused by diabetes. Synergy may also be involved. As an example, the protection against free-radical damage is more efficient with both approaches than by the actions of either alone.

Some types of cellular damage caused by free radicals can be repaired by enzymes. Enzymes are special proteins that speed specific chemical reactions along. Some enzymes are made solely to repair damage to cells caused by free radicals and by high levels of blood sugar.

Antioxidants reduce the damage that free radicals do to cell components and to the enzymes that repair cells, by reducing oxygen modification of proteins. However, without the additional protection of chromium picolinate and insulin working together to prevent the formation of sugar-damaged enzymes, these enzymes will become inactive and unable to repair cell damage. Even though the repair enzymes are protected by antioxidant nutrients, the damage caused by high blood sugar levels quickly becomes significant.

Chromium picolinate reduces the protein damage that high blood sugar levels cause without causing these levels to drop sharply. It works by helping insulin control blood sugar fluctuations so that proteins are not exposed to short bursts of high blood sugar levels.

When chromium picolinate prevents the damage from blood sugar, and antioxidants protect against free radicals, then the minor damage that does occur can be repaired by the still-functioning enzymes. The result is the cell is protected and the body does not become damaged and thereby "one cell older."

In 1970, my research was sufficiently advanced that it was granted patents in several countries.[3] My main contribution was the recognition of the biological synergism of the antioxidant nutrients. The synergism approach made the antioxidant approach practical for humans. Dr. Denham Harman had developed the free-radical theory of aging, but he was working with single nutrients that had to be taken in very large — and impractical — amounts.[4] My unified theory of aging was reported in *Chemical & Engineering News* on October 26, 1970.

Those who chose to follow my advice in 1970 are more than 20 years ahead of those just starting today to use antioxidant nutrient supplements. If you choose to follow my latest advice, and if it is on target as I believe it is, you will be many years ahead of your skeptical friends who decide to wait until there is conclusive scientific support.

When making such a decision, you must look at the benefit-to-risk ratio. There are major benefits in optimizing your chromium intake with chromium picolinate beyond the immense benefit of greater longevity.

Chromium picolinate has already been proven to lower harmful LDL-cholesterol, improve good HDL-cholesterol, and help insulin control blood sugar levels. Many studies have shown that chromium picolinate helps increase our lean tissue while reducing our fat tissue. In other words, chromium picolinate helps build muscle while reducing fat.

As for risks, there are none in following this approach. There are no practical toxicity problems. The only persons who should take precautions are diabetics. Diabetics can improve their blood sugar levels so rapidly that their blood sugar level could fall too low if they neglect to monitor it and adjust their insulin intake. I suggest that diabetics consult a physician when taking chromium picolinate.

The only real risk is *not* to follow this approach. I personally cannot afford to wait 20 or 30 years for all the data to come in. Can you?

There is a prudent time when there are enough data available to accurately predict what the result will be. In the remainder of this book, I will share the available data with you, and you can decide for yourself.

REFERENCES

1. Plans for a large-scale study of possible retardation of the human aging process. Passwater, Richard A. *The Gerontologist* 10(3):11,28 (1970).

2. Human Aging Research, Part II. Passwater, R. A. and Welker, P.A. *American Laboratory* 3(5):21-26 (1971); also *International Laboratory* 37-40 (July/August 1971).

3. US 39140; Germany P-21-24-972,9; Great Britain 16047/71

4. The free-radical theory of aging. Harman, Denham. *J. Gerontol.* 11:298-300 (1956).

2

The Aging Process

ONE AFTERNOON in the late 1970s I was standing in line at the Air and Space Museum in Washington to get tickets for the wonderful movie, "To Fly." The line wound around the new Skylab exhibit, which was showing our latest space technology.

A father and his young son were standing behind me. The son said, "Dad — that looks brand-new! You said museums were for old things." His father replied, "Son, some things are old in a short time. Some can even be old before they are finished."

I realized that I wanted to be that way, not to be "finished" before I grow old. I want to still be doing things when I get old, to get older without getting *old*.

But, it would be no fun to live longer unless my family and friends would also live longer and better. Therefore, I am writing this to help us all live better longer. To understand how chromium picolinate may help us put more life into our years, it will be helpful if you understand some basic facts about the aging process and how long we live.

The measure of how *long* we live is called the lifespan. We have no scientific measurement of how *well* we live; we just refer to an undefined "quality of life." A better quality of life implies having the capability of being physically and mentally active and having an absence of disease. Living better longer means that we should be just as active physically and mentally in our older years as we normally are in our middle years. This means being a "young senior." The ideal is to be a member of the "young old" group until just a short time before our necessary decline at the end of our lifespan.

Unfortunately, too many people are "older than their years"; they are members of the "aged old" group with incapacitating illness and accelerated aging, although they existed and suffered for many long years. Looking at lifespan tables doesn't show the difference. The goal is to live with more vitality for more years.

Lifespan

Let's look at the progress that we have been making in lifespan and see if we can determine how much of that progress was made by secondary factors and how much, if any, was made by slowing the aging process. Normally, when we speak of lifespan of a species or group of humans, we are considering the "average" number of years lived by everyone in the group. Since the maximum lifespan is more or less fixed, changes in average lifespan reflect changes in the lifespans of the young far more than the old.

There is a definite genetic contribution to lifespan. After all, desert creosote bushes are said to live for 10,000 years and redwood trees may live 4,000 to 5,000 years, but mice rarely live more than three years.

Records indicate that early man lived an average of 15 years, about the same as cats or sheep. For the Neanderthal, that was barely long enough to allow for species reproduction and caring for the young. During the period from 400 BC to 600 AD, Greeks and Romans averaged about 30 years, about the same as a lion or horse. By the Middle Ages, the lifespan in Europe averaged about 31 to 33 years, and even in 1750 in England, it was still only 35 years. One hundred years later in 1850, in England the average lifespan had climbed to about 40 years.

In 1900 in the U.S.A., the average lifespan was 47 years. Today, it is about 75 years.

As we had better access to purer water, food preservation and distribution improved, and physicians learned to wash their hands to reduce infectious diarrhea and childbirth fever, fewer died young. In the 1940s, miracle drugs — the antibiotics — helped control infectious diseases. Vaccines help control diphtheria, whooping cough, typhoid and polio. Smallpox, once the world's most dreaded plague, was completely eradicated by 1977. All of these helped increase the average lifespan by allowing the younger to live longer.

Table 2.1 shows how the average lifespan has increased in this country since 1900.

Table 2.1. Increase in average human lifespan since 1900.

Year	Average Lifespan
1900	47.3
1910	50.0
1920	54.1
1930	59.7
1940	62.9
1950	68.2
1960	69.7
1970	70.9
1980	73.7
1986	74.9

Table 2.2 lists the ten leading causes of death in 1860, 1900 and 1970. You can readily see how curtailing the infectious diseases has increased our average lifespan. However, even as we learn to curtail heart disease and cancer, the average lifespan will not increase beyond about 90 years. Only when we learn to slow the aging process itself can we expect to see significant further

improvement. This will be discussed more fully in the next chapter.

When you look at the gains in life expectancy for those who have already achieved 75 years of age, there has been very little progress over the years. In 1900, the life expectancy of the average 75-year-old was about nine years, and in 1980 it was about ten years.

Table 2.2. Leading causes of death.

Rank	1860	1900	1970
1	Tuberculosis	Pneumonia, flu	Heart disease
2	Diarrhea, Enteritis	Tuberculosis	Cancer
3	Cholera	Diarrhea, enteritis	Stroke
4	Pneumonia, flu	Heart disease	Pneumonia, flu
5	Infantile convulsions	Nephritis	Non-vehicle accidents, suicide
6	Stroke	Accidents	Vehicle accidents
7	Diphtheria, croup	Stroke	Diseases of early infancy
8	Dysentery	Diseases of early infancy	Diabetes
9	Scarlet fever	Cancer	Arterios-clerosis
10	Nephritis	Diphtheria	Cirrhosis

From all indications, at the present rate of progress, the average lifespan in the U.S. is going to top out at about 85 years.probably around 2050, and the maximum lifespan is still going to be about 115 to 120 years. But, what if new technology or knowledge changes the current rate of progress? There is no evidence that the body has an internal aging clock or genetic factor to make it fall apart at 85 or 120 years of age. There is good evidence that our neurons could survive 200 or more years, if their support system continued to function properly.

The existing laboratory animal and human clinical evidence suggests that chromium picolinate will increase our average lifespan due to several factors. A companion of its effects with other of other approaches is summarized in Table 2.3. But, will chromium picolinate actually slow the aging process? To answer that question, we should discuss the aging process itself.

Table 2.3. Effects of different approaches on lifespan and cholesterol levels.

	Increase in Lifespan	Effect on Cholesterol	Reference
Exercise	10 months	Significant lowering	1
Low-fat Diet	Probably 3 to 10 months	5 percent	2-5 lowering
Antioxidants	Probably 10 to 15 years	Protective	6, 7
Chromium Picolinate	Possible 10 to 15 years or more	Significant lowering	8

The Aging Process

The American Medical Association's Committee on Aging studied the problem of human aging for more than a decade and concluded that not one physical or mental condition was directly attributable to the passage of time alone. Some of the so-called diseases of old age — such as arthritis, high blood pressure or heart disease — are prevalent in the young as well as the old. Other diseases, such as osteoporosis or benign prostate disease, are the result of lengthy periods of undernutrition, not the result of time alone. Well-nourished persons do not develop such maladies even in their nineties. What exactly is aging, then, and what are its causes?

Aging can best be described as the process that reduces the number of healthy cells in the body. Although we have noted the increase of some enzymes in the body and the decrease of others, the most striking factor in the aging process is the body's loss of reserve to respond to a challenge to its status quo (homeostasis).

What causes the body to lose its capacity to respond to a threat? The disappearance of cells from organs and tissues means that there is less of an organ or body system to produce what is needed to counter the threat. The body loses its ability to reproduce some of its cells and, as cells are destroyed, they are not always replaced. One by one, the cells disappear until there isn't enough of the working tissue left to adequately handle the challenge.

A good illustrative metaphor is that of an old theater marquee that consists of thousands of light bulbs. The light bulbs are turned on and off to produce a message. As time goes by, the light bulbs burn out one by one until the message can no longer be read. Like so many lights on the marquee, the cells die, eventually shutting off the entire network.

An example of how the body loses reserves with aging is that fasting blood glucose (blood sugar) levels remain fairly constant throughout life in the healthy individual. However, the glucose tolerance measurement, which measures the reserve capacity of the body to respond to the stress of drinking a large amount of a sugar solution, shows a loss of response with age. The same holds true concerning the recovery mechanisms of other systems. An older person in the best aerobic shape will breathe harder doing the same work than a younger person in the best aerobic shape does, and the older person will take longer to return to a normal breathing rate.

Dr. Charles Barrows of the Gerontology Center wrote in 1970, "We know, from animal studies, that death of cells in certain organs and tissues accompanies age. We can count the cells and note the reduction." It is as great as 55 percent in the skeletal muscles of extremely old rats. We know also that the weight of a 75-year-old man's brain is less than that of the brain of a 35-year-old, due to cell loss. This cell loss is greatest in nerve, muscle, kidney, and glands, which accounts for the gradual loss (about 0.6 percent per year on average) of their functions.

In addition to the loss of cells, there is a stiffening of tissues. In the early 1960s, it was this stiffening or linking together of cells that I concentrated on. The linking together of molecules, cells and tissues was studied as part of the cross-linking theory of aging that was postulated by Dr. Johan Bjorksten. I was studying how the ultraviolet energy of the sun and various chemicals in our diet could fuse molecules together in such a way as to link tissues together and cause their stiffening. Dr. Bjorksten was looking for enzymes that would undo this cross-linking and rejuvenate the body. By the mid-1960s it became apparent to me that free radicals could produce cross-linking as well as other damage. Later, I learned that blood sugar could react with body proteins to change their chemical and physical characteristics. As I mentioned in the first chapter, these proteins are called "sugar-damaged" proteins, and they cause aging in several ways, primarily by cross-linking and stiffening tissues and organs.

Together, the loss of cells and the linking or stiffening of tissues age our bodies. Clinical studies show that the maximal physiological capacities of most organ systems decline progressively and inexorably after age 30.[9] Although no specific disease is due to time alone, the gradual loss of visual and auditory acuity with age is common knowledge. Heart, lung and kidney efficiency declines as a linear function of age. The heart becomes stiffer and less efficient as a pump, while arteries lose elasticity and offer greater resistance to blood flow. This, in turn, decreases blood flow to most organs, including the kidneys, which thus become less efficient as filters. The maximal capacity of the stiffened lungs to exchange gases (fresh oxygen in, stale carbon dioxide out) declines.

The stiffening of skin is very noticeable as we age. In fact, a common test of the "age" of our skin is to pinch the skin on the back of a hand and time how long it takes to return to its original position. Skin that has been excessively aged by sunlight is stiff and takes longer to return to its normal position than younger, more flexible skin.

You can prove to yourself, unless you are a nudist, that this is not a result of time passing by, but of exposure to sunlight, by comparing the skin on the back of hands or necks to that on the buttocks. The exposed skin on the hands and neck behaves much differently from skin that has been protected by clothing. This difference doesn't exist in young children because they haven't had years of sun exposure to their skin. Because there is this difference in older people and not in the young, we say this difference is the result of aging. It is not due to time alone, however.

The aging process also impairs our immune system, primarily owing to decreased effectiveness of so-called cellular immunity, which is crucial for protection against viruses and tumors. Wound healing takes longer in an older person. A scraped knee heals in a day or so in a young child, but the same abrasion might persist for weeks in an elderly person.

The aged brain has lost a large percentage of cells in several key neural pathways; therefore reaction time is longer, learning becomes less efficient, and short-term memory becomes less reliable.

Of course, through exercise and improved nutrition, people at any age can increase their physiological capacities — but the *maximal* capacity they can achieve by their best efforts will inevitably decline with increasing age.

The greatly diminished physiological capacities of each organ system mean that old people are far more likely to die if subjected to stresses such as infection, accidental injury or environmental factors such as extreme cold or heat, and even air pollution.

The stability of the living system becomes progressively impaired by chemical reactions, not the passage of time. If we can control the rate of these deleterious reactions, we can control the aging process. Slowing the aging process has a very dramatic effect on the lifespan — much more so than the effect of eliminating diseases such as heart disease and cancer. Eliminating all cancer would increase the average lifespan by only about two years.[9] Total prevention of all coronary heart disease would increase the average lifespan by about seven years.

And even if disease prevention were able to increase the average lifespan by, say, two decades, how many people would want to live their last 30 or 40 years free of major disease, but severely functionally impaired and dependent on daily nursing care?

It is clear that, in order for major increases in lifespan to be both achievable and desirable, the aging process itself must be slowed.

We have the tools to do that now. Although the aging process appears very complex when viewed as a group of specific chemical reactions, we can simplify matters by concentrating primarily on the loss of information in the molecules responsible for reproducing the body's proteins. Free radicals and glycation are the responsible culprits. Glycation is the modification of a protein by the addition of a sugar molecule. We have already discussed free radicals and we will discuss glycation in the next chapter. Antioxidant nutrients protect against free radicals while chromium protects against glycation.

After studying the aging process for more than 30 years, it is my opinion that what we have come to recognize as the signs of aging are the result of two basic processes. One is the fundamental aging process itself, and the second is a process determined by secondary factors — that is, environmental factors such as each individual's lifestyle and nutrition. The combined effects of both processes determine our apparent age, i.e., the age others assume us to be.

These secondary factors typically cause aging signs to appear ten to 20 years earlier than they would under ideal circumstances. There is abundant evidence that many signs of old age are due solely to secondary factors and are not even related to aging. Older people simply have had more time and opportunity to abuse their bodies through suboptimal nutrition and poor lifestyles.

In Chapter 4, we will examine the evidence that chromium picolinate extends the lifespans of laboratory animals and also reduces the formation of sugar-damaged proteins that cause aging of all species. Thus, we will see where chromium picolinate may both slow the aging process and increase lifespan. But first, let's discuss how blood sugar fluctuations damage proteins, and how that damage causes aging. Then we can examine how slowing the production of sugar-damaged protein with chromium picolinate may slow the aging process. The next chapter deals with both processes.

REFERENCES

1. The association of changes in physical-activity level and other lifestyle characteristics with mortality among men. Paffenbarger, R. S.; Hyde, R. T.; Wing, A. L.; Lee, I. M.; Jung, D. L. and Kampert, J. B. *New Engl. J. Med.* 328(8):538-45 (Feb. 25, 1993).

2. Expected gains in life expectancy from various coronary heart disease risk factor modifications. Tsevat, J.; Weinstein, M. C.; Williams, L. W.; Tosteson, A. N. and Goldman, L. *Circulation* 83(4):1194-1201 (April 1991).

3. The cholesterol myth. Moore, Thomas J. *Atlantic Monthly* 37-57 (September 1989).

4. *Heart Failure.* Moore, Thomas J. Random House, NY (1989).

5. Effects of coronary risk reduction on the pattern of mortality. Rose, Geoffrey and Shipley, Martin. *Lancet* 335(8684):275-7 (February 3, 1990).

6. The human aging process. Passwater, Richard A. and Welker, Paul. *American Laboratory* 3(4):36-40 (April 1971).

7. *The New Supernutrition.* Passwater, Richard A. Pocket Books, NY (1991).

8. Chromium picolinate increases longevity. Evans, Gary and Meyer, L. *Age* 15:134 (1992).

9. *Principles of Mammalian Aging.* Kohn, R. R. Prentice-Hall, Englewood Cliffs, NJ (1978).

3

Slowing the Aging Process: Calorie Restriction

NOW THAT we understand what aging is, let's see how we can slow aging and increase our healthy lifespan. In this chapter we will examine lines of research that lead to practical results. The first approach is well supported by scientific evidence, but, unfortunately, requires a severe cutback in the amount of food that we eat. Calorie restriction does result in extended youth and longer life, but most people don't want to pay such a high price.

The second approach uses the information gained from the first approach, and shows us how chromium picolinate can produce virtually all of the benefits of calorie restriction without actually restricting your diet. Let's look at the two approaches and then examine the evidence that shows chromium picolinate increasing the average lifespan of animals by more than one-third. For comparison, a 36 percent increase would extend the average human lifespan from about 75 years to over 100 years.

The Calorie Restriction Approach

Now remember, calorie restriction is not the approach that I am excited about. This information is discussed so that you can see how calorie restriction and chromium picolinate have a common mechanism and produce the same result. The big difference is that calorie restriction requires extreme sacrifice and chromium picolinate doesn't.

You may have heard of the benefits of calorie restriction thanks to Dr. Roy Walford's books, *Maximum Lifespan* and

The 120-Year Diet.[1,2] This approach started in the 1930s with research by Dr. Clive McCay. In the early years of the Depression, Dr. McCay and his colleagues at Cornell University were wrestling with an issue that was then a lively topic of scientific controversy: How does the growth rate of animals correlate with their longevity?

Dr. McCay had noted that species with longer periods of growth and maturation tended to live longer than those who mature more rapidly. He was curious to see if individuals within a species followed the same pattern. So he decided to divide a colony of rats randomly into several groups and systematically slow the growth of some groups by underfeeding them.

One group of rats had unlimited access to food 24 hours a day and could eat as they desired. Scientists refer to this eating pattern as "ad-libitum feeding" or "ad-lib" for short. Two other groups were allowed to grow in a "stair-step" fashion. For two or three months they would be given just enough food each day to maintain a stable weight, then they would be given a greater amount of food for a while, until they achieved a predetermined weight gain.

At the end of the first year, the ad-lib fed rats were three times heavier than the food-restricted rats. The food fed to the restricted rats had ample protein and was rich in vitamins and minerals, so the rats were well-nourished and were deficient only in calories.

After two years plus a month, Dr. McCay allowed half of the rats fed the restricted calorie diet to eat ad-lib. They rapidly gained size and weight.

When the last rat in Dr. McCay's experiment had died, he analyzed the longevity of the various groups. The average lifespan of the male rats was decidedly greater in the calorie-restricted groups. The ad-lib fed rats lived an average of 483 days. However, the rats that were calorie-restricted all of their lives lived for an average of 894 days, while those who were calorie-restricted for a little more than two years and then allowed to eat ad-lib lived an average of 820 days. In addition, Dr. McCay noted that one-sixth of the restricted males had lived longer than 1,200 days — a lifespan longer than Dr. McCay could find reported in the scientific literature for any rat.

For the female rats, the results weren't as clear-cut — possibly because several of the restricted-diet females died at a very early age during a heat wave. (This was during the Depression, before the days of air-conditioned laboratories.) When these early deaths due to the heat wave are eliminated from the experiment, the results are similar to those for the male rats. A significant proportion of the female rats fed a calorie-restricted diet exceeded the age of 1,200 days, including one female Methuselah who lived 1,421 days — which is almost four years. Dr. McCay concluded, "These data indicate clearly that some factor tended to promote longevity in the calorie-restricted groups."[3]

Dr. McCay's findings were published in 1935 in the *Journal of Nutrition*.[3] In effect, this classic research article inaugurated the science of life extension. Nearly 60 years of subsequent research, using many different strains of rodents, have confirmed Dr. McCay's fundamental observation that calorie restriction tends to increase both average and maximal lifespan.[4,5]

Confirming Studies

More recent studies have used climate-controlled barrier facilities which protect laboratory animals from germs, thus eliminating the possibility that epidemics would skew the average lifespans of the animals. Calorie restriction is now typically achieved by feeding the restricted-diet animals 20 to 40 percent fewer calories each day than the amount that ad-lib fed animals eat. Calorie-restricted animals typically have both average and maximal lifespans 20 to 50 percent greater than ad-lib fed animals.

It is important to note that the calorie-restricted diets are enriched with vitamins and minerals so that all diets are equal in vitamin and mineral content. Thus, these studies demonstrate the longevity effect of calorie restriction alone and do not involve malnutrition or differences due to vitamin or mineral content.

The aging and cross-linking of collagen, the main protein in skin, can be more accurately measured than the simple skin pinch test described in Chapter 2. Scientists can accurately measure the strength of the collagen fibers and how long the collagen fibers take to be digested by an enzyme. By measuring these parameters, the amount of collagen cross-linking can be determined. In 1959, Czech scientists were the first to demonstrate that calorie restriction slowed the aging of skin in laboratory animals.[6] They measured the strength of the collagen fibers.

These findings were confirmed and extended by the Australian gerontologist Dr. Arthur Everitt. Dr. Everitt found that in rats receiving one-third fewer calories throughout their lives, the collagen in their skin at 900 days was equivalent to the collagen in the skin of 600-day-old rats which were allowed to eat ad-lib.[7]

Collagen also accumulates in the organs of aging animals. Dr. Zurba Deyl and colleagues in Prague reported that this collagen accumulation commenced at about 20 months in ad-lib fed rats, whereas in calorie-restricted rats, it did not begin until 32 months.[8]

Calorie restriction retards the cross-linking and accumulation of collagen in aging animals. More generally, this shows that calorie restriction slows the crucial age-related changes that make tissues stiffer and drier.

Calorie restriction slows the fundamental aging process in many other ways. Aging animals experience an increase in pituitary hormones, a decrease in bone mass, and many other chemical and cellular changes that can be measured and hence studied. Calorie restriction has been shown to slow *all* of the changes studied.[9,10]

Of particular interest are the positive effects of calorie restriction on the immune system. Calorie restriction slows the decrease in size of the thymus. The thymus is a small gland-like organ located just behind the sternum of the chest that is crucial for the production of an important immune system component, the T-lymphocytes. Normally as we age, the thymus shrinks and is replaced by fat and collagen, and our immune system loses a proportional ability to make the T-lymphocytes. Thus calorie restricted animals have improved immune systems as measured by cellular immunity and other immune parameters.[11]

Like the thymus, the pineal gland is a small organ that undergoes gradual degeneration with increasing age. Located at the base of the brain, the pineal produces hormones such as melatonin which regulate the activity of a crucial control center in the brain called the hypothalamus. Some scientists believe that regression of the pineal gland acts as a pacesetter for aging, and recent studies show that properly timed administration of melatonin or pineal extracts can prolong lifespan and boost immunity.[12,13] Not surprisingly, calorie restriction has been found to preserve the structures and function of the pineal gland in aging rats.[14,15]

Calorie restriction also has a positive effect on brain function and behavior. As animals age, their spontaneous activity declines; aging calorie-restricted rats are much more active than ad-lib fed rats. Aging mice take considerably longer than younger mice to master a maze. At 31 to 35 months, the maze-learning ability of calorie-restricted mice is more similar to that of far younger mice than to that of their ad-lib fed contemporaries. Calorie-restricted mice also show improved performance in coordination tests.[16]

These findings establish that calorie restriction acts at a very fundamental level to genuinely slow the aging process. Calorie restriction doesn't just prevent disease to yield "healthy" senile, decrepit animals. At an age when most ad-lib fed rats are dying of senile disorders, calorie restricted rats *act younger, look younger, and by objective physiological standards of aging, actually are younger.*

The prevention or delay of age-related disease in calorie-restriced animals can be viewed as just one of the many benefits of the "anti-aging" effect of calorie restriction.

Slowing Aging Prevents Diseases

Not surprisingly, autopsy studies show that calorie restriction prevents or retards the onset of several fatal diseases.[17,18] For example, severe kidney disease (chronic nephropathy) is a major cause of death in rats, and most rats which achieve a normal lifespan are found to have significant kidney disease when autopsied. In contrast, calorie restriction almost totally prevents kidney disease and eliminates it as a significant cause of death. Atrophy and fibrosis of the heart muscle lead to congestive heart failure, which is another leading cause of death in rats, but not in calorie-restricted rats.

You may be thinking that this doesn't apply to humans because we die chiefly of cancer and heart diseases such as acute myocardial infarction and coronary thrombosis, and not so much from kidney disease and congestive heart failure. Well, if we live long enough and avoid the coronary artery diseases and cancer, which are largely antioxidant-deficiency diseases, then we tend to die of congestive heart disease and kidney disease. The goal of this book is to help you avoid both the coronary artery diseases and most of the other "old age" diseases. Chromium picolinate has an important role in achieving both goals.

The fact that calorie restriction decreases the incidence of these diseases is pertinent to us, but remember, I am going to show you how the same benefits can be obtained without resorting to calorie restriction. Now let's get back to the effect calorie restriction has on preventing diseases.

In studies conducted at the University of Texas Health Sciences Center in San Antonio, Drs. Edward Masoro and Byung Pal Yu and their colleagues found that the age of onset of early heart damage rose from 18 months in the ad-lib fed rats to 30 months in the calorie-restricted groups. Similarly, the onset of most tumors is delayed by calorie restriction.[18]

Calorie restriction also delays or prevents autoimmune diseases such as kidney damage (nephropathy) and arterial inflammation (periarteritis).

Disease prevention, as important as it is, is by no means the most exciting benefit of calorie restriction. If the only benefit of calorie restriction were disease prevention, you would merely grow old in "good health" (free of disease), but you would still suffer the infirmities of old age and die of cell-depleted, aged tissues unable to overcome insults or challenges to the body. I emphasize again that calorie-restricted animals look and act more like younger animals. Underfeeding calories while providing the optimal amounts of vitamins and minerals appears to slow the primary aging process, retarding the rate at which physiological functions decline.

Calorie restriction produces all of these benefits, yet we don't hear too much about it. That is probably because it is virtually impossible to willingly go through life eating less than 1,500 calories each day. However, we can achieve most of the benefits of caloric restriction without even testing our will power. The important information is not that calorie restriction works, but what calorie restriction does to produce these benefits.

The good news is that we have learned how calorie restriction works. Calorie restriction is believed to have a small positive effect on the hypothalamus in the brain, but it works chiefly because it reduces the amount of protein damage caused by blood sugar fluctuations. This protein damage causes proteins to link together and tissues to stiffen and lose their flexibility. The evidence is that chromium picolinate also reduces this formation of "sugar-damaged" protein. Sugar-damaged proteins and oxygen-damaged proteins lead to the aging of our tissues, as will be discussed in the next chapter.

REFERENCES

1. *Maximum Lifespan.* Walford, Roy L. Norton & Co., NY (1983).

2. *The One hundred and Twenty Year Diet: How to double your vital years* Walford, Roy L. Simon & Schuster, NY (1987).

3. The effect of retarded growth upon the length of life span and upon the ultimate body size. McCay, C. M.; Crowell, M. F. and Maynard, L. A. *J. Nutr.* 10:63-79 (1935).

4. Food restriction in rodents: An evaluation of its role in the study of aging. Masoro, E. J. *J. Gerontol.* 43:B59-B64 (1988).

5. *The Retardation of Aging and Disease by Dietary Restriction.* Weindruch, R. and Walford, R. L.Charles C Thomas, Springfield, IL (1988).

6. The influence of aging and undernutrition on chemical contractility and relaxation of collagen fibers in rats. Chvapil, M. and Hruza, Z. *Gerontologia* 3:241-52 (1959).

7. Food intake, growth and the ageing of collagen in rat tail tendon. Everitt, A. V. *Gerontologia* 17:98-104 (1971).

8. The effect of food deprivation on collagen accumulation. Deyl, Z.; Juricova, M.; Rosmus, J. and Adam, M. *Exp. Geront.* 6:383-90 (1971).

9. Retardation of the aging process in rats by food restriction. Masoro, E. J.; Shimokawa, I. and Yu, B. P. *Ann. NY Acad. Sci.* 621:337-52 (1991).

10. Food restriction research: Past and present status. Yu, B. P. *Rev. Biol. Res. Aging* 4:349-71 (1990).

11. Effect of calorie restriction on the production and responsiveness to interleukin 2 in (NZBXZW) f-1 mice. Jung, L. K. L.; Palladino, M. A.; Calvano, S.; et al. *Clin. Immunol. Immunopathol.* 25:295-301 (1982).

12. The pineal control of aging. The effects of melatonin and pineal grafting on the survival of older mice. Pierpaoli, W.; Dall'ara, A.; Pedrinis, E. and Regelson, W. *Ann. NY Acad. Sci.* 621:291-313 (1991).

13. The pineal peptides: Interaction with indoles and the role in aging and cancer. Anisimov, V. N.; Bondarenko, L. A.; Khavinson, V. Kh. and Morozov, V. G. *Neuroendocrin. Lett.* 11:235 (1989).

14. Pineal gland structure and respiration as affected by age and hypocaloric diet. Walker, R. F.; McMahon, K. M. and Pivorun, E. B. *Exp. Geront.* 13:91-99 (1978).

15. Food restriction retards aging of the pineal gland. Stokkan, K. A.; Reiter, R. J.; Nonaka, K. O.; et al. *Brain Res.* 545:66-72 (1991).

16. Dietary restriction benefits learning and motor performance of aged mice. Ingram, D. K.; Weindruch, R.; Spangler, E. L.; et al. *J. Gerontol.* 42:78-81 (1987).

17. Nutrition and longevity in the rat. II. Longevity and onset of disease with different levels of food intake. Berg, B. N. and Simms, H. S. *J. Nutr.* 71:255-63 (1960).

18. Life span study of SPF Fischer 344 male rats fed ad libitum or restricted diets: Longevity, growth, lean body mass and disease. Yu, B. P.; Masoro, E. J.; Murata, I., et al. *J. Gerontol.* 37:130-141 (1982).

4

Glycation:
The Link Between Calorie Restriction
And Chromium Picolinate

ASIDE from Dr. Roy Walford, I don't know of any one who admits to trying to slow aging by severely restricting his calories. I know of a few scientists who eat very little, and I suspect that they are trying calorie restriction as a health benefit, if not to slow their aging. But they won't even admit that.

You would have to be very, very motivated to restrict calories sufficiently to slow aging. Table 4.1 shows the number of calories required to maintain constant weight, and the number required for calorie restriction. As your weight drops because you are not maintaining constant weight, you have to adjust your calories downward. In his book *Maximum Lifespan,* Dr. Walford recommended 1,500 calories daily. This is the amount that I calculate for a 130-pound person. However, I am not sure at what weight you will stabilize 1,500 calories a day. I don't believe that the energy calculations presented in the 10th edition of *Recommended Dietary Allowances* apply at that intake.[1]

It is most unlikely that many people could succeed in voluntarily reducing their daily calorie intakes by one-third or more throughout their lives — just look at the dismal long-term success rates of most calorie-counting reducing diet programs. Choosing low-fat foods — the most effective technique for long-term weight control — may reduce calorie consumption a bit, but most people on low-fat diets eat an increased volume of food so that the calorie intake doesn't drop dramatically.

Table 4.1. Calorie requirements for weight maintenance and calorie-restricted diets.

Body weight (pounds)	Calories to maintain constant weight (average activity)	Maximum calories for a calorie-restricted diet to slow aging
130	2,200	1,455
145	2,550	1,700
160	2,900	1,935
175	3,250	2,170

Unfortunately, calorie restriction per se may have very limited practical applicability in humans. But if we understand how calorie restriction works to extend longevity, we can develop *practical* measures to replicate its benefits.

As you may recall, Dr. Clive McCay first attempted calorie restriction to test the theory that delaying growth and development would prolong longevity. Fortunately, many studies have come along to prove that restricting calories and development *after* growth is complete is virtually as successful in extending youth as is lifelong caloric restriction.

Can you imagine if we had to restrict calories in our hungry, growing kids and then end up with more decades of teen-agers? Wow! Fortunately, the mechanism is not halting growth! Retardation of growth has *nothing* to do with the life extension effect of calorie restriction.

We can also eliminate the possibility that reduced intake of any one dietary component, such as protein, fat, or minerals, is the factor that produces the results. Scientists tried ad-lib diets that were very low in fat or protein or minerals, only to find that they did not slow the aging process.

So far we have eliminated growth retardation and individual dietary components as the mechanism of life extension. Another theory was that calorie restriction worked because it reduced the metabolic rate. It is thought that metabolism slows down during reduced-calorie diets. The "reduced metabolism" theory was the most popular hypothesis until Dr. Edward Masoro's group at the University of Texas Health Sciences Center made a surprising discovery. After an initial period of several weeks during which calorie-restricted animals lose weight or fail to gain weight, they reach an equilibrium at which their metabolic rate is equal to or even slightly higher than that of ad lib–fed rats.[2]

This is possible — despite a substantially reduced daily caloric intake — because chronically calorie-restricted animals have far less lean mass than their ad lib–fed counterparts; typically, they weigh half as much. So, once equilibrium is reached, their caloric intake and their metabolic rate *per unit lean mass* is not less than that of far heavier ad lib–fed animals. So much for the "reduced metabolism" theory of calorie restriction.

To me, losing lean muscle is not worth slowing the aging process. There still is a way of obtaining the benefits of calorie restriction without losing lean muscle tissue or restricting calories. Chromium picolinate helps build muscle, reduce fat, and in limited animal studies, has extended average and maximum lifespans. And as we will see shortly, the common mechanism is reducing the formation of sugar-damaged proteins. The scientific name for producing sugar-damaged proteins is "glycation."

However, before we can establish that the mechanism important in aging is glycation, we must rule out some other possibilities. Several studies conducted in the 1970s suggested that body temperature was slightly lower in calorie-restricted animals. Since all biochemical reactions proceed more slowly at reduced temperatures, and since low ambient temperatures tend to increase the lifespan of cold-blooded animals, it was reasonable indeed to suspect that reduced body temperature had something to do with the longevity effect of calorie restriction. Harvard studies reported in 1984, however, that lower body temperature was not the mechanism that produced the benefits of calorie restriction.[3]

Calorie-restricted animals have far less body fat than ad lib–fed animals. Could reduced body fat be the key? Researchers assessed this possibility by studying a special strain of mouse that has a strong tendency to obesity. The mice, which normally become massively obese, were calorie-restricted so that their body weights were kept comparable to those of ad lib–fed from a closely related but non-obese genetic strain. Because of their genetic defect, the calorie-restricted "obese" mice had substantially more body fat than the ad lib–fed mice but they also lived much longer despite their greater fat mass.[4] This, as well as other observations, indicate that low body fat is not responsible for the longevity effect of calorie restriction.[5]

Clearly, the field of gerontology is littered with bright ideas about calorie restriction that haven't stood up to experimental scrutiny. Is there light at the end of the tunnel? In fact, there *are* some recent observations that bring us to the answer for much, but not quite all, of the puzzle.

Glycation: What is it and what harm does it do?

In 1988, Dr. Edward Masoro and colleagues reported that blood sugar (blood glucose) levels were about 11 percent lower in calorie-restricted animals.[6] The reason that this piqued his interest is that previously, scientists — notably Dr. Anthony Cerami of Rockefeller University — had shown that increased levels of blood sugar could accelerate the aging process.

This idea arose from attempts to explain the secondary complications and accelerated tissue aging associated with diabetes, a disorder where average blood sugar levels are far above normal. Scientists discovered that the collagen of comparatively young diabetics was as rigid and as highly cross-linked as that of extremely old people.

Dr. Robert Kohn and colleagues at Case Western Reserve University were studying tissues from healthy persons and diabetics, when they noted a problem. They used a technique that was highly accurate in estimating the age of healthy persons, but was very inaccurate for diabetics. In 14 nondiabetics their estimates, based on tissue samples and without seeing the individuals, were remarkably accurate, not off by more than a few years. But, they were spectacularly wrong in the three juvenile-onset (type I) diabetics who were in their 30s and 40s. The tissues from these diabetics tested out to be those of 80- to 100-year-olds.[8]

Clearly, collagen ages much more rapidly in diabetics. The functional consequences of this have been demonstrated clinically. In young diabetics, the lungs and arteries have greatly reduced elasticity, similar to those of very old people.[9,10]

Spurred by these and related findings, scientists discovered that blood sugar (glucose) and other sugars called reducing sugars, such as fructose and ribose, could react spontaneously — without the need for enzymes — with collagen and other proteins to form cross-linked, sugar-damaged proteins.[11,12]

The rate of sugar modification of proteins is proportional to sugar concentration, so it is evident that the hyperglycemia (high blood sugar) of diabetics leads to an increased rate of collagen cross-linking. A good analogy is that the cross-linking of proteins is like putting hand-cuffs on the proteins so that they can't move about freely, as they are designed to do. It is like stapling them together and then to an immovable object.

As I mentioned earlier, the process of forming these sugar damaged proteins is called "glycation." The actual sugar-damaged proteins and complex derivatives of glucose themselves are called "advanced glycosylation end products," or "AGEs" for short.[13] That's not a bad acronym, as "AGEs" lead to an "aged" body at an early age. AGEs are yellowish-brown fluorescent structures. The process can be compared to the browning reaction in toast and sliced apples. The formation rate of AGEs increases as both the blood sugar level and the length of time it is raised increase.

The spontaneous reaction of sugar with tissue proteins such as collagen and myelin is responsible for accelerated tissue aging in diabetics; it is believed to be responsible for kidney damage and is involved in the atherosclerosis process; these last are both common complications of diabetes.[13] Dr. Anthony Cerami then postulated that glycation reactions also play a role in the normal aging of tissue. He gathered more data which resulted in his "glycation hypothesis of aging.[7,14–16]

Recent studies show that diabetics as well as aging animals do indeed have increased concentrations of AGEs in their collagen.[12,13,17] Of related interest is the fact that average blood sugar levels tend to rise with increasing age owing to the fact that for unknown reasons the tissues of aging animals (including humans) become less sensitive to the actions of insulin.[18] It is not just a loss of reserve due to aging and the loss of tissue, but it directly involves the interaction of insulin and the tissues themselves.

The roles of oxygen-damaged protein and sugar-damaged protein definitely explain many of the secondary aging effects and some of the primary aging process. Nevertheless, they fall far short of offering a complete explanation of the entire aging process. Despite these reservations, it appears likely that, other factors being equal, high blood sugar levels, and also wide fluctuations in blood sugar levels, increase the cross-linking of collagen and other important proteins. Conversely, maintaining precise blood sugar control at the optimal level throughout life should result in tissues that are "young for their age."

The link between calorie restriction and glycation prevention is that there are fewer sugar-damaged proteins and AGEs formed in both. While the calorie-restriction approach is impractical for most of us, the glycation theory of aging has given rise to a recent study that should prove to have profound *practical* implications for health and longevity. In the next chapter, we will discuss how a simple supplement, chromium picolinate, reduces glycation and extends the lifespans of laboratory animals.

REFERENCES

1. *Recommended Dietary Allowances,* 10th ed. National Research Council (U.S.), Subcommittee on the Tenth Edition of the RDAs. Food and Nutrition Board. National Academy Press, Washington, D.C. (1989).

2. Action of food restriction in delaying the aging process. Masoro, E. J.; Yu, B. P. and Bertrand, H. A. *Proc. Natl. Acad. Sci.* 79:4239-41 (1982).

3. Effect of dietary restriction and stress on body temperature in rats. Volicer, L.; West, C. and Greene, L. *J. Gerontol.* 39:178-82 (1984).

4. Effects of food restriction on aging: Separation of food intake and adiposity. Harrison, D. E.; Archer, J. R. and Astle, C. M. *Proc. Natl. Acad. Sci.* 81:827-35 (1984).

5. Changes in adipose mass and cellularity through the adult life of rats fed ad libitum or a life prolonging restricted diet. Bertrand, H. A.; Lynd, F. T.; Masoro, E. J. and Yu, B. P. *J. Gerontol.* 35:827-35 (1980).

6. Evidence for the glycation hypothesis of aging from the food-restricted rodent model. Masoro, E. J.; Katz, M. S. and McMahan, C. A. *J. Gerontol.* 44:B20-B22 (1989).

7. Glucose and aging. Cerami, A.; Vlassara, H. and Brownlee, M. *Scientific American* 90-6 (May 1987).

8. Apparent accelerated aging of human collagen in diabetes mellitus. Hamlin, C. R.; Kohn, R. R. and Luschin, J. H. *Diabetes* 24:902-4 (1975).

9. Arterial pulse waves and velocity and systolic time intervals in diabetic children. Pillsbury, H. C.; Hung, W.; Kyle, M. D. and Freis, E. D. *Amer. Heart J.* 87:783-90 (1974).

10. Abnormal lung elasticity in juvenile diabetes mellitus. Schuyler, M. R.; Niewoehner, D. E.; Inkley, S. R. and Kohn, R. *Amer. Rev. Resp. Dis.* 113:37-41 (1976).

11. Collagen aging in vitro by nonenzymatic glycosylation and browning.Kohn, R. R.; Cerami, A. and Monnier, V. M. *Diabetes* 33:57-9 (1984).

12. Nonenzymatic glycation of collagen in aging and diabetes. Reiser, K. M. *Proc. Soc. Exp. Med.* 196:17-29 (1991).

13. Advanced glycosylation end products in tissue and the biochemical basis of diabetic complications. Brownlee, M.; Cerami, A. and Vlassara, H. *New Engl. J. Med.* 318:1315-21 (1988),

14. In vitro and in vivo reactions of nucleic acids with reducing sugars. Lee, A. T. and Cerami, A. *Mutat. Res.* 238(3):185-91 (1990).

15. Nonenzymatic glycosylation of DNA by reducing sugars. Lee, A. T. and Cerami, A. *Prog. Clin. Biol. Res.* 304:291-9 (1989).

16. Advanced glycosylation products quench nitric oxide and mediate defective endothelium-dependent vasodilation in experimental diabetes. Bucala, R.; Tracey, K. J. and Cerami, A. *J. Clin. Invest.* 87(2):432-8 (1991).

17. Increased glycation and pigmentation of collagen in aged and young parabiotic rats and mice. Deyl, Z.; Butenko, G. M.; Hausmann, J.; et al. *Mech. Ageing Develop.* 55:39-47 (1990).

18. Mechanisms of age-related glucose intolerance. Jackson, R. A. *Diabetes Care* 13(Suppl 2):9-19 (1990).

5

The Evidence for Chromium Picolinate

THE PURPOSE in discussing the aging process and how it can be slowed by calorie restriction, and to a lesser degree, by antioxidant nutrients, was to provide the background necessary to understand how chromium picolinate works. Chromium picolinate reduces the production of sugar-damaged proteins which age our bodies. We discussed in the previous chapter how glycation aged body tissues. Now we are ready to discuss how chromium picolinate reduces glycation and, as demonstrated in a laboratory study, increases average and maximal lifespans.

Chromium picolinate is a safe and biologically effective form of the trace mineral chromium. Its effectiveness in extending life, lowering cholesterol, building muscle, and reducing body fat has been established by scientific studies which will be discussed in this chapter and those that follow. Some forms of chromium, such as chromic chloride, have been found to be inefficient and have not been shown scientifically to produce the benefits demonstrated in many studies using chromium picolinate.

Chromium was shown to be an essential nutrient for humans in the 1950s by Drs. Klaus Schwarz and Walter Mertz when they were together at the National Institutes of Health.[1] To date, the sole documented physiological function of chromium is to help insulin do its job.[2] The function of insulin is to help nutrients such as glucose and amino acids enter and be used by cells. Somehow, insulin permits the passage of these nutrients from the blood and through the cell membranes into the cell interior, but it cannot function without biologically active chromium.

We know that some biologically active chromium compounds help insulin function, but the nature of these compounds still under investigation by scientists. We don't know exactly what they are or how they work. The biologically active chromium compound — or compounds — is sometimes called the glucose tolerance factor, or GTF. However, no compounds having this activity have been isolated under conditions stable enough for further study, and there is no general scientific agreement as to what the structure of the so-called glucose tolerance factor might be.

I wrote a booklet about GTF chromium in 1982, and there has been little significant progress to report since then.[3] But we do know that some chromium compounds, such as chromium picolinate or those found in brewer's yeast, do work, directly or indirectly through intermediaries while others do not significantly aid insulin function. We do know that chromium picolinate leads to improved insulin function. The presence of picolinic acid in yeast may account for its biological activity.

One researcher, Dr. Gary Evans of Bemidji State University in Minnesota, believes that chromium picolinate itself is the elusive glucose tolerance factor. Dr. Evans believes that chromium picolinate, as an intact molecule, alters the fluidity of cell membranes so that insulin functions better.[4]

Severe chromium deficiency, whether in humans or other animals, leads to a dramatic impairment of insulin function, resulting in symptoms similar to diabetes. As mentioned earlier, one of the chief functions of insulin is to promote the uptake of blood sugar (blood glucose) by muscles and many other tissues. If insulin does not function effectively, blood sugar remains abnormally elevated after a meal. This is glucose intolerance. In overt diabetics, insulin action is even more profoundly impaired; production of additional glucose by the liver cannot be suppressed and blood sugar levels remain high even after an overnight fast.

With diabetes, the problem can be not enough insulin production or, when there is enough insulin to normally do the job, the insulin isn't working effectively. The so-called type I or "juvenile" diabetes results from damage to the pancreas that impairs its ability to produce insulin. The much more common form of diabetes — non-insulin dependent diabetes mellitus (NIDDM) (also called type II or "adult-onset" diabetes) — results from a failure of the body's tissues to respond effectively to insulin. With NIDDM, blood insulin levels are often normal or even elevated.

Today, due to the prevalence of high-fat, refined diets and sedentary lifestyles, many people have insulin sensitivity problems, even though they don't have actual NIDDM. Their tissues become resistant to insulin. In most of these individuals, the pancreas compensates by secreting more insulin so that severe glucose intolerance or diabetes is averted.[5] However, high blood levels of insulin are not beneficial. They have been linked to increased risk of heart disease and other illnesses.[6-10] Finally, chromium nutrition is drawing appropriate interest as scientists realize that insulin resistance poses grave health dangers.

Studies showing chromium picolinate increases lifespan

Dr. Evans took note of the glycation theory of aging and decided it would be interesting to see whether lifelong feeding of chromium picolinate had any effect on longevity. He and L. Meyer took 30 weanling rats and separated them randomly into three groups of ten. Each group received the same amount of chromium in their diets, but one group received its chromium in the form of chromium picolinate, another group received chromic chloride, while the third group received a chromium/niacin complex.

After 300 and 1,000 days, the researchers measured the blood sugar and glycosylated hemoglobin levels of the laboratory animals. ("Glycosylated" "glucosylated" and "glycated" are synonymous terms, with each being associated with different items according to their historical usage.) The glycosylated hemoglobin measures the amount of glycation of the red blood cells. This gives a clinical measure of the time-integrated average of blood sugar level over the preceding several weeks, rather than just a single point in time value.

(I found that glycosylated hemoglobin was a much more meaningful indicator than blood sugar measurements when I was studying the effect of high-chromium brewer's yeast on diabetic mice in the early 1980s. This measurement gives a much truer idea of the sugar–protein interactions over a period of time than the momentary measurement of single points in time that blood sugar levels indicate.)

Aside from these measurements, the laboratory animals were not bothered, and were allowed to live out their lives eating as much food as they wished. The researchers kept track of the age at death as each animal died from natural causes.

Four years later, the results were reported at the October 1992 meeting of the American Aging Association in San Francisco.[11] These findings are summarized in Table 5.1. At 300 days, both blood glucose and glycosylated hemoglobin were slightly reduced in the chromium picolinate group relative to the two other groups. At 1,000 days, the disparities were dramatic. Blood sugar was 20 percent lower and glycosylated hemoglobin was over 50 percent lower in the chromium picolinate group than in the other two groups.

The big surprise was the difference in mortality between the chromium picolinate group and the others. The median lifespan of the chromium picolinate group was 45 months, compared to only 33 months in the other two groups. That is an improvement of 36 percent. To put this lifespan improvement in perspective, if the average U.S. male lifespan is taken to be 75 years, a 36 percent improvement would result in an average lifespan of 102 years.

Table 5.1. Results of feeding chromium picolinate to rats.

	Chromium picolinate group	Chromic chloride and chromium/ niacin complex group
Average lifespan	45 months	33 months
Improvement in average lifespan	36 %	—
Longest-lived survivor	48 months	41 months
improvement in maximum lifespan (over controls)	17%	—
Improvement in maximum lifespan (over species history)	14%	—

Looking at the ages of the longest-living survivors in the three groups, the longest-surviving rat in the chromium picolinate group was 48 months of age, while neither of the other two groups had survivors exceeding 41 months of age.

Scientists are trained to be skeptics, so they must look closely at the results. They must consider the possibility that the results were statistical flukes. Two follow-up studies are in progress, but it will take several years before other scientists can confirm these results. What can we deduce in the meantime?

The closeness of the average and maximal lifespans of the chromium picolinate group is a very positive sign.

This indicates that the results were not skewed by one or two very long-lived animals as a fluke. It also indicates that more of the animals were approaching their maximal lifespan, which became the limiting factor. The adequacy of the diet and environmental considerations was demonstrated by the fact that the longest-lived controls very closely matched their species historical maximum of 42 months.[12] More than half of the chromium picolinate group animals lived beyond the 45 months, which in itself exceeds the species historical maximum. The numbers do indeed indicate that the chromium picolinate exerted a true and remarkable effect.

Another factor which enhances the credibility of these results is that Dr. Evans in fact conducted two long-term feeding studies with chromium picolinate. The second study was a toxicologic study to evaluate whether life-long feeding of chromium picolinate might produce any adverse effects.[13]

In the other study, designed primarily to look at safety, weanling rats received 0, 0.25, 0.5, 1.0 or 5.0 parts per million of their diet as chromium, in the form of chromium picolinate. When the rats reached 30 months of age, Dr. Evans noticed a curious effect: 9 of the 20 rats in the lower potency groups had died, whereas only one of the 30 in the higher potency groups (0.5 ppm chromium or higher) had died.

Since this was a toxicologic study, all of these rats were sacrificed soon after 30 months of age for autopsy. Thus, the average lifespan and maximal lifespans could not be determined. However, the results were certainly consistent with a longevity effect for chromium picolinate.

Incidentally, no adverse effects were found on autopsy in any of the groups, and it is notable that no adverse effects have been observed in any of the clinical studies to date with chromium picolinate.

But Dr. Evans was not the first scientist to report a longevity effect in a toxicologic study with chromium. Back in the 1930s, Dr. John Byerrum reported on toxicologic tests with an unstable chromium salt. Dr. Walter Mertz discussed this evidence in a review in 1969.[14]

We now know that calorie restriction lowers average insulin levels, as does chromium picolinate. We can also see how both calorie restriction and chromium picolinate may similarly affect the hypothalamus and pineal gland. We also know that a drug that improves insulin sensitivity also improves lifespan. There is little reasonable doubt that insulin sensitization improves health and lifespan, and that chromium picolinate reduces the production of sugar-damaged proteins that age the body. Let us now turn to how chromium picolinate helps protect us against major diseases and, as a bonus, improves our physiques by building lean tissues and reducing fat tissues.

REFERENCES

1. Chromium (III) and the glucose tolerance factor. Schwarz, Klaus and Mertz, Walter. *Arch. Biochem.* 55:292-3 (1959).

2. Chromium in human nutrition. Offenbacher, E. G. and Pi-Sunyer, F. X. *Ann. Rev. Nutr.* 8:543-63 (1988).

3. *GTF Chromium.* Passwater, Richard A. Keats Publishing, Inc., New Canaan, CT (1982).

4. Composition and biological activity of chromium-pyridine carboxylate complexes. Evans, Gary W. and Pouchnik, D. J. *J. Inorg. Biochem.* 49:177-87 (1993).

5. Variations in insulin-stimulated glucose uptake in healthy individuals with normal glucose tolerance. Hollenbeck, C. and Reaven, G. M. *J. Clin. Endocrinol. Metab.* 64:1169-73 (1987).

6. Hyperinsulinaemia is a predictor of non-insulin-dependent diabetes mellitus. Zimmet, P., Dowse, G. and Bennett, P. *Diabete Metabolisme* 17:101-8 (1988).

7. Role of insulin resistance in human disease. Reaven, G.M. *Diabetes* 37: 1595-1607 (1988).

8. Resistance to insulin-stimulated-glucose uptake in patients with hypertension. Shen, D.C.; Shieh, S.M.; Fuh, M.T.; et al. *J. Clin. Endocrinol. Metab.* 66: 580-3 (1988).

9. Risk factors for coronary artery disease in healthy persons with hyperinsulinemia and normal glucose tolerance. Zavaroni, I.; Bonora, E.; Pagliara, M.; et al. *New Engl. J. Med.* 320: 702-6 (1989).

10. A multifaceted syndrome responsible for NIDDM, obesity, hypertension, dyslipidemia, and atherosclerotic cardiovascular disease. DeFronzo, R.A. and Ferrannini, E. *Diabetes Care* 14:173-94 (1991).

11. Chromium picolinate increases longevity. Evans, G.W. and Meyer, L. *Age* 15: 134 (1992).

12. Striatal dopamine, sexual activity and lifespan. Longevity of rats treated with deprenyl. Knoll, J.; Dallo, J. and Yen, T. T. *Life Sciences* 45:525-31 (1989).

13. Chromium picolinate is an efficacious and safe supplement. Evans, Gary W. *Int. J. Sport Nutr.* 3:117-9 (1993).

14. Chromium occurrence and function in biological systems. Mertz, Walter. *Physiol. Rev.* 49:163-239 (1969).

6

Heart Disease

SEVERAL times I have mentioned that chromium picolinate not only appears to slow aging, it has also been shown to increase the lifespan by reducing the risk of killer diseases such as heart disease. Studies show that if blood levels of chromium reach optimal levels, heart disease is extremely unlikely.[1,2] Even more exciting is that studies also show that chromium can eradicate existing cholesterol deposits in the arteries.[3-5] Indeed there are many studies showing that improving chromium intake directly slashes the rate of heart disease, and these studies have been reviewed in the scientific literature.[6,7] Many other studies show chromium deficiencies increase the rate of heart disease.[7,9] Several studies show that increasing dietary chromium reduces the amount of cholesterol in the blood[10-13], and conversely, that decreasing dietary chromium raises blood cholesterol.[14]

Chromium helps keep the arteries deposit-free by increasing the body's ability to remove cholesterol. Cholesterol is carried to cells by a carrier called low-density lipoprotein (LDL). The left-over and unneeded cholesterol is carried back to the liver by a carrier called high-density lipoprotein (HDL). HDL is a very efficient cholesterol scavenger, and when you make more HDL, more cholesterol will be captured by HDL. When all of the cholesterol excess produced by the liver is captured, the HDL even draws cholesterol out of any deposits that may exist in the arteries. Chromium increases HDL production.[15]

Regression of Cholesterol Deposits Is Possible

Let's look more closely at the tremendously exciting studies that show that chromium can reverse atherosclerosis. But before we look at the regression studies, let's examine a background study conducted by researchers at Ohio State University and the Medical College of Ohio.

The researchers measured the chromium concentrations in 32 patients who were presented for angiography, the procedure where a radio-opaque dye is injected into the coronary arteries and a movie is taken via fluoroscopy. Only the subjects whose chromium levels were above 5.5 micrograms per liter of blood were free of coronary heart disease. Those with coronary heart disease had much lower blood chromium concentrations than those with healthy arteries.[1]

A later study showed an even more striking relationship between blood chromium levels and the incidence of cholesterol deposits. Patients suffering from the symptoms of coronary artery disease were referred to the Division of Cardiology in Bordeaux-Gradignan, France. The patients were then grouped according to the number of coronary arteries significantly blocked by cholesterol deposits or in medical terms, plaque.

The researchers concluded that "an upper limit for chromium could exist beyond which the likelihood of developing coronary artery disease or heart disease is improbable."[2]

Now, let's consider the study that demonstrated that, at least in animals, cholesterol deposits can be dissolved away. Rabbits were fed a diet that produced cholesterol deposits in their arteries. After eight weeks, the presence of the cholesterol deposits was confirmed, and the rabbits were then fed a normal diet. The rabbits were then divided into two groups, with one group given a daily chromium supplement while the remaining group was given a placebo. After 30 weeks, their aortas were examined. Those not receiving the chromium had 50 percent more cholesterol deposits than those receiving the chromium supplement. The researchers concluded, "The results show a significant effect of chromium on the regression of cholesterol-induced atherosclerotic plaques in rabbits."[4]

This research group expanded upon their study in 1991. Again they concluded that "animals fed the chromium supplement showed greater regression of established cholesterol-induced plaques [than animals] fed placebos. The regression appeared independent of blood lipid values."[5]

Chromium Picolinate Lowers Cholesterol and Increases HDL

As mentioned earlier, the reason that chromium picolinate can dissolve cholesterol deposits from arteries is that it increases the amount of the cholesterol scavenger called HDL that circulates in the blood. High-density lipoprotein is a particlelike aggregate of compounds assembled by the liver to seek out, pick up and carry cholesterol back to the liver. It can even scavenge cholesterol from cholesterol deposits in arteries.

The better the ratio of HDL to LDL, the better the arteries. It is not as important to know how high your cholesterol level is as it is to know your HDL/LDL ratio.

Chromium picolinate lowers the number of LDL particles and the amount of LDL cholesterol, while increasing the number of HDL particles and the amount of HDL cholesterol. Thus, chromium picolinate improves your HDL/LDL ratio and clears your arteries.

Researchers led by Dr. Raymond Press of the Mercy Hospital and Medical Center of San Diego, studied LDL, HDL and cholesterol levels in 28 healthy volunteers.[11] Earlier studies had shown that chromium increased

HDL by 23 percent (Mossop, 1983) and 17 percent (Riales,1981), lowered LDL by 17 percent (Riales, 1981), and lowered total cholesterol by 10 percent (Offenbacher, 1980), 14 percent (Schroeder, 1968) and 36 percent (Canfield, 1979). The San Diego researchers wanted to study chromium picolinate using the latest procedures.

In the double-blind cross-over study led by Dr. Press, the volunteers were randomly divided into two groups by a researcher not otherwise participating in the study. Each group took a daily supplement, but neither the volunteers nor the researchers knew which supplement was being taken by any volunteer during the study. One group received 200 micrograms of chromium in the form of chromium picolinate daily for 42 days, while the other group received a placebo. The volunteers then abstained from taking their supplement for 14 days.

After this rest, the supplements were changed. The first group now received the supplement that the second group had taken during the first part of the study, and vice versa. The volunteers took the new supplement for 42 days. This is called a cross-over, and it eliminates many study variables, since each person is both a control and a test subject.

When the study was completed and the code broken, the researchers found that those who were first given the chromium picolinate had lower cholesterol, lower LDL-cholesterol and lower apolipoprotein B (which is used to form LDL). They also had higher HDL-cholesterol and apolipoprotein A-1 (which is used to form HDL). During this time, those receiving the placebo had no significant changes in their cholesterol, lipoproteins or apolipoproteins.

When the capsules were switched, those who were receiving the placebo and now were taking the chromium picolinate had the same improvements that the first group had when they took the chromium picolinate. And strikingly, those who had benefited from the chromium picolinate during the first part of the study, and were now receiving the placebo, saw their improvements fade as their chromium levels fell.

In a similar study with diabetic subjects, chromium picolinate was shown to decrease total cholesterol by 8 percent and LDL-cholesterol by 6 percent in just six weeks.[11]

Dr. Geoffrey Gordon, also of San Diego, combined chromium picolinate, the B-vitamin niacin and dietary advice to achieve a 24 percent reduction in total cholesterol, 27 percent reduction in LDLcholesterol, 43 percent reduction in triglycerides and an improvement in HDL/LDL ratio in ten patients with high cholesterol levels.[12]

Dr. John Roeback of the University of North Carolina found that a daily supplement of high-chromium yeast (600 micrograms of chromium) raised HDL levels by 16 percent, even when the patients were also taking blood-pressure medication that normally lowers HDL.[16]

Now that we have established chromium picolinate's protective role against heart disease, let's take a look at its possible role in protection against cancer.

REFERENCES

1. Serum chromium and angiographically determined coronary artery disease. Newman, Howard A. I.; Leighton, Richard F.; Lanese, Richard R. and Freedland, Neil A. *Clin. Chem.* 24:541-4 (1978).

2. Low plasma chromium in patients with coronary artery and heart disease. Simonoff, Monique; Llabador, Y.; Hamon, C.; et al. *Biolog. Trace Element Res.* 6:431-9 (September-October 1984).

3. Cineangiographically determined coronary artery disease and plasma chromium level for 150 subjects. Simonoff, Monique; Llabador, Y. and Simonoff, G. N. *Nucl. Instr. Meth.* 231, (1984).

4. The effect of chromium on established atherosclerotic plaques in rabbits. Abraham, Abraham S.; Sonnenblick, Moshe; Eini, Maya; Shemesh, Ovadiah and Batt, Aharon P. *Amer. J. Clin. Nutr.* 33:2294-8 (November 1980).

5. Chromium and cholesterol-induced atherosclerosis in rabbits. Abraham, Abraham S.; Brooks, B. and Enlath, U. *Ann. Nutr. Metab.* 35:203-7 (1991).

6. Vascular prostacyclin may be reduced in diabetes in man. Johnson, M. et al. *Lancet* I:325 (1979).

7. Trace minerals and atherosclerosis. Mertz, Walter. *Fed. Proc.* 41:2807-12 (1982).

8. Chromium deficiency as a factor in atherosclerosis. Schroeder, Henry A.; Nason, B. S. and Tipton, Isabel H. *J. Chron. Dis.* 23:123-42 (1970).

9. Chromium deficiency and cardiovascular risk. Simonoff, Monique. *Cardiovas. Res.* 18:591-6 (1984).

10. Chromium metabolism in man and biochemical effects. Doisy, R. J.; Streetan, D. H. P.; Freeberg, J. M.; et al. In: *Trace Elements in Human Health and Disease,* Vol. II. Prard and Oberleas, (eds.) (1976).

11. The effect of chromium picolinate on serum cholesterol and apolipoprotein fractions in human subjects. Press, Raymond I., Geller, Jack and Evans, Gary W. *West. J. Med.* 152:41-5 (1990).

12. An easy and inexpensive way to lower cholesterol? Gordon, Geoffrey B. *West. J. Med.* 154:3 (March 1991).

13. Serum cholesterol reduction by chromium in hypercholesterolemic rats. Staub, H., Reussner, G. and Thiessen, R. *Science* 166:746-7 (1969).

14. The role of chromium in mammalian nutrition. Schroeder, Henry A. *Amer. J. Clin. Nutr.* 21:230-11 (1968).

15. Effect of chromium chloride supplementation on glucose tolerance and serum lipids including high-density lipoproteins of adult men. Riales, R. and Albrink, M. *Amer. J. Clin. Nutr.* 34:2670-8 (1981).

16. Effect of chromium supplementation on serum high-density lipoprotein cholesterol levels in men taking beta-blockers. Roeback, John R.; Hla, Khin Mae; Chambless, Lloyd E. and Fletcher, Robert H. *Ann. Intern. Med.* 115(12):917-24 (December 15, 1991).

7

The Aging Immune System and Cancer

THE RISK and incidence of cancer increases with age. Part of the explanation is obvious; many cancers take several years — even decades — to develop. Also one's likelihood of exposure to any given cause of cancer increases with time, and one's "body burden" of carcinogens increases with time. However, a young and healthy person is protected against the cancer process by his or her immune system. It is only when the immune system is overwhelmed by massive and constant exposure to a carcinogen, such as in the everyday working environment, or the immune system is impaired by undernutrition or *aging* that cancer develops.

If we could maintain the same healthy immune system of our youth, virtually the only persons developing cancer would be those who had inherited genetic defects in their immune system. "Cancer" is a group of about 180 diseases involving the body's cells characterized by a multi-step process involving initiation, promotion, progression, cancer, and metastasis. The immune system has the potential to halt the cancer process at each and every step.

Initiation occurs when free radicals or AGEs react with DNA in such a way that, when the cell divides to accomplish growth or replacement, the new cell is a mutant. The damaged DNA is normally repaired by enzymes in healthy young persons, but as people age, they normally lose about one percent of their capacity to repair DNA each year.[1] Their DNA repair enzymes, which are proteins, become sugar-damaged or oxygen-damaged. This damage to the repair enzymes can be reduced by better blood sugar regulation with chromium picolinate, and by better free-radical control with antioxidants.

A second factor is that cells normally control their replication via sensors on the cell membranes. These sensors, which are proteins, can be damaged by glycation or by free radicals. When the replication sensors are sugar-damaged or oxygen-damaged, they lose their ability to recognize the proximity of "like" (identical cell type) cells. Normally, the recognition of "like" cells in close proximity shuts down the cell replication (mitosis). If these protein sensors are damaged, then the cell growth can go out of control.

The immune system can detect mutated cells and destroy them, unless the immune system is impaired. It is believed that people normally develop mutated cells on a regular basis, but their immune system destroys them before a tumor develops. With a high frequency of mutation normally occurring, small declines in immune system performance over the years become significant.

Support for the premise that reduced glycation yields a lower incidence of cancer comes from the calorie-restriction approach. It is well established that fats can be tumor promoters, but their role in cancer is more complex. Fats are a concentrated source of calories, and calories are important in the cancer process. More research is needed to separate the effects of excess body fat and dietary fat on cancer risk, but there is good support for reduced glycation being a significant factor.

In 1943, Drs. P. S. Lavik and C. A. Baumann investigated the influences of dietary fat and total calories on the incidence of cancer and found that laboratory animals fed a high-fat, low-calorie diet produced 48 percent fewer tumors than those fed a low-fat, high-calorie diet.[2] Recently, Dr. David Kritchevsky of the Wistar Institute in Philadelphia and Dr. D. Albanes of the National Cancer Institute reviewed more than 80 studies and found that diets high in calories but low in fat were distinctly more carcinogenic than those low in calories but high in fat.[3-5]

Dr. Kritchevsky and colleagues have shown that the incidence of both colon and mammary tumors is significantly lower in rats whose caloric intake is 40 percent lower than that of ad lib–fed controls.[6,7] The fat content of the calorie-restricted diet was more than double that of the ad-lib diet. Dr. Kritchevsky's group then studied the effects of progressive caloric restriction in laboratory animals restricted in calories by 10, 20, 30 or 40 percent. Tumor incidence was reduced (compared to the ad lib–fed controls) by 0, 33, 50 and 92 percent.[8] Several investigators have found that the earlier calorie restriction is begun, the greater the inhibition of tumor growth.[9-11] In fact, the conformation of the beneficial effect of calorie restriction on cancer can be traced back to 1909.[12]

In Chapter 4, we saw that calorie restriction worked largely by reducing the production of sugar-damaged proteins and/or AGEs. It is very probable that the same results can be achieved by optimal chromium intake. It remains to be seen if chromium picolinate supplements will reduce the incidence of cancer. However, to me, it seems very prudent to reduce both sugar-damaged proteins and oxygen-damaged proteins with optimal intake of chromium and antioxidant nutrients.

REFERENCES

1. DNA repair and aging in basal cell carcinoma: A molecular epidemiology study. Wei, Q.; Matanoski, G. M.; Farmer, E. R.; Hedayati, M. A. and Grossman, L. *Proc. Natl. Acad. Sci.* 90(4):1614-8 (February 15, 1993).

2. Further studies of tumor promoting action of fat. Lavik, P. S. and Baumann, C. A. *Cancer Res.* 3:749-56 (1943).

3. Calorie restriction and experimental tumorigenesis. Kritchevsky, David. *Nutrition Today* 28(1):25-7 (1993).

4. Total calories, body weight and tumor incidence in mice. Albanes, D. *Cancer Res.* 47:1987-92 (1987).

5. Caloric intake, body weight, and cancer: A review. Albanes, D. *Nutr. Cancer* 9(4):199-217 (1987).

6. Dietary fat versus caloric content in initiation and promotion of dimethylbenz(a)anthracene-induced mammary tumorigenesis in rats. Kritchevsky, D.; Weber, M. M. and Klurfeld, D. M. *Cancer Res.* 44:3174-7 (1984).

7. Inhibition of chemically-induced mammary and colon tumor promotion by caloric restriction in rats fed increased dietary fat. Klurfeld, D. M.; Weber, M. M. and Kritchevsky, D. *Cancer Res.* 47:2759-62 (1987)

8. Determination of the degree of energy restriction necessary to reduce DMBA-induced mammary tumorigenesis in rats during the promotion phase. Klurfeld, D. M.; Welch, C. B.; Davis, M. J. and Kritchevsky, D. *J. Nutr.* 119:286-91 (1989).

9. Dietary restriction in mice beginning at one year of age: effect on life span and spontaneous cancer incidence. Weindruch, R. and Walford, R. L. *Science* 215:1415-8 (1982).

10. Lasting influence of early caloric restriction on prevalence of neoplasms in the rat. Ross, M. H. and Bras, G. *J. Natl. Cancer Inst.* 47:1095-1113 (1971).

11. Nutrition and cancer. Tannebaum, A. In: Hornburger, F., ed. *The Physiopathology of Cancer.* Hoeber-Harper, Inc., New York, (1959).

12. Beziehungen zwischen ernahrung und tumorwachstum. Moreschi, C. Z. *fur Immunitatsforsch.* 2:651-75 (1909).

8

Preventing and Controlling Diabetes

UNFORTUNATELY, diabetes not only ages the body prematurely, it shortens the lifespan as well. The good news is that clinical studies have shown that chromium picolinate reduces the damage caused by diabetes by (a) helping insulin work to control blood sugar levels and (b) reducing the production of sugar-damaged proteins.[1-4] We discussed this at some length in Chapter 4. In this chapter we will look at the clinical studies specifically addressing diabetes itself.

Researchers at the Mercy Hospital and Medical Center of San Diego studied the effect of chromium picolinate on "type II" diabetes (non-insulin dependent diabetes mellitus or NIDDM). Dr. Raymond Press and colleagues measured the fasting blood sugar levels and glycosylated hemoglobin levels in NIDDM patients.

Glycosylated hemoglobin provides better information about blood sugar, over a long period of time, than merely measuring the blood sugar level itself at various times. With diabetes, the blood sugar and insulin levels can fluctuate wildly. Knowing the level at any instant tells little about what happened before and after that particular measurement.

As a red blood cell circulates, it combines some of the glucose in the bloodstream with its own content of hemoglobin to form glycosylated hemoglobin in an irreversible reaction. The amount of glycosylated hemoglobin formed and stored by a red blood cell depends on the amount of glucose available to it during the cell's

120-day lifespan. This fact makes the measurement of glycosylated hemoglobin a valuable indicator of the blood sugar condition over an extended period. This is a "time-averaged" indicator rather than a transient value.

The researchers found that 200 micrograms of chromium (as chromium picolinate) reduced fasting blood sugar levels by 18 percent and glycosylated hemoglobin levels by 10 percent in just six weeks.[5,6]

In a small preliminary study of American Chippewa Indians with NIDDM, fasting blood sugar levels decreased markedly after two weeks of supplementation with chromium picolinate. After eight weeks of supplementation, fasting blood sugar levels decreased by 32.6 percent from a mean of 258 mg/dL to a mean of 168 mg/dL.[17]

CAUTION: Chromium picolinate is so effective that diabetics should not take chromium picolinate unless they are going to carefully monitor their blood sugar level under the supervision of a physician.

Looking and Feeling Younger

The next chapter will discuss how chromium picolinate helps build lean tissue (muscle) and reduce body fat.

REFERENCES

1. Impaired intravenous glucose tolerance as an early sign of dietary necrotic liver degeneration. Mertz, Walter and Schwarz, Klaus. *Arch. Biochem. Biophys.* 56:504-6 (1955).

2. Chromium metabolism and its role in disease processes in man. Anderson, Richard A. *Clin. Physiol. Biochem.* 4:31 (1986).

3. Use of the artificial beta cell (ABC) in the assessment of peripheral insulin sensitivity: Effect of chromium supplementation in diabetic patients. Elias, Alan N.; Grossman, Marshall K. and Valenta, Lubomir J. *Gen. Pharmac.* 15(6):535-9 (1984).

4. Chromium may prevent Type II diabetes onset. Anderson, Richard A. and Polansky, Marilyn M. *Sci. News* 137:214 (April 7, 1990).

5. The effect of chromium picolinate on serum cholesterol and apolipoprotein fractions in human subjects. Press, Raymond I.; Geller, Jack and Evans, Gary W. *West. J. Med.* 152:41-5 (1990).

6. The effect of chromium picolinate on insulin controlled parameters in humans. Evans, Gary W. *Intern. J. Biosocial Med. Res.* 11(2):163-80 (1989).

7. An inexpensive, convenient adjunct for the treatment of diabetes. Evans, Gary W. *West. J. Med.* 155:549 (November 1991).

8. Chromium supplementation of human subjects: Effects on glucose, insulin and lipid parameters. Anderson, Richard A.; Polansky, Marilyn M.; Bryden, Noella A.; et al. *Metabolism* 32:894-9 (1983).

9

Paring Away Body Fat

EXCESS body fat is not consistent with a youthful lifestyle. The good news is that chromium picolinate helps us look younger and trimmer while increasing lifespan. Many scientists were surprised to learn that chromium picolinate was found repeatedly to reduce body fat even without dieting or exercising. This has even been confirmed in several animal studies, so the results can't be attributed to psychological factors.

However, chromium picolinate can produce gradual but steady and persistent loss of body fat. When the positive benefit of chromium picolinate is complemented, as it should be, by a reduction in dietary fat and an increase in exercise, the fat loss is proportionally accelerated.

Now, I know how difficult it is to diet and to lose weight; I have had experience with many thousands of dieters. As a consultant to Weight Loss International, Inc. in the early 1970s, I developed two diet programs that helped many dieters, and chromium was stressed in both.[1,2] However, chromium picolinate was not available then.

It is not unreasonable to expect that chromium picolinate will help dieters lose weight for several reasons. However, the studies that show that chromium picolinate in and of itself would produce gradual weight loss were surprising. Let's look at some of the reasons why chromium could be expected to help chromium-deficient dieters. Remember that *nine out of ten people* do not get the minimum amount of chromium recommended.

Chromium deficiency increases fat production because it slows the burning of food for energy. The non-fuel food calories are then converted to fat and stored in fat tissues.

As will be explained shortly, chromium deficiency upsets the appetite control center and can cause a "false hunger." This is when hunger persists even after the blood sugar level is high enough to stop hunger ordinarily, but because insulin is inefficient in chromium deficiency, the blood sugar doesn't get into the brain cells that control the appetite. Chromium deficiency can also contribute to wild swings in blood sugar levels that can result in serious mood changes.

The results of early research suggested that chromium picolinate by itself — in the absence of increased exercise — could increase fat loss. Studies were then designed to test this possibility. By the end of 1991, three other studies were completed, all supporting the premise that chromium picolinate does indeed decrease body fat and build muscle even without dieting or increased exercise.[3,5]

One study was done at a prominent weight-loss clinic in San Antonio, Texas under the direction of Dr. Gilbert Kaats. Volunteers consumed two nutritional drinks each day and were not asked to change their food intake or exercise activity, although some may have done so. Some of the drinks contained no chromium picolinate, some contained 200 micrograms of chromium picolinate and others, 400 micrograms of chromium picolinate. Neither the doctors nor the volunteers knew how much chromium picolinate was in their drinks until after the study. Others had prepared the nutritional drinks, coded them and kept the codes secret until after the study. Then the code was released and the results compiled.

After 72 days, the group receiving no chromium picolinate had essentially no fat loss or muscle gain. However, the groups receiving chromium picolinate did have significant improvements which averaged a loss of 4.2 pounds of fat and a gain of 1.4 pounds of muscle. That's a net improvement of 5.6 pounds. We can call this improvement a net enhancement of the physique.

The results were best in the older volunteers, which is not surprising, since chromium deficiency increases with age. Those taking 400 micrograms of chromium picolinate daily averaged a 27 percent better response than those taking 200 micrograms of chromium picolinate daily.

To prove that the results weren't psychological or induced by bias, the studies were repeated with animals. One study at Louisiana State University found that chromium picolinate (but not inorganic chromic chloride) reduced fat measured at the tenth rib by 21 percent and increased muscle 7 percent.[4] A second study at Virginia Polytechnical Institute confirmed that feeding chromium picolinate reduced back fat while increasing muscle (pork chop) size.[5]

Tips on Faster Fat Loss
In addition to taking chromium picolinate, reduce your fat intake, drink more water and increase exercise to speed results. Drink at least eight glasses of water and/or clear fluids every day. A lot of what you sense as being hunger is really a thirst. Your body may be telling you that you need more water — and since you do not drink enough water by itself, your body will signal you to eat more food, which may be 50 to 90 percent water. Getting water in food, however, also increases the number of calories consumed.

For a week, keep a diary of what you eat. You will find that you eat more snacks than you thought. Use this information to reduce your snacks, especially bedtime snacks. Keep track of the total number of grams of fat you eat each day. Try to cut at least 15 grams of fat from your daily diet. Eventually try to limit your fat calories to 25 percent of your total dietary intake. You can do this without reducing your total calories by substituting high-carbohydrate foods for high-fat foods. The 25/25 diet — 25 percent fat, 25 grams of fiber — works well for trimming your body, and it is a general, all-purpose healthy diet.

Dietary fat, according to recent research, does not appear to reduce hunger in proportion to calorie value and it is quickly stored in fat tissue. Fat is not taken into the glucostats in the appetite control center. As mentioned earlier, carbohydrates turn off hunger via the glucostats of the appetite control center; fat does not.

Also, chromium and insulin work together after a high carbohydrate meal to temporarily increase metabolism in what is known as "carbohydrate-mediated thermogenesis." This is why equal-calorie meals do not always produce the same amount of body fat. High-carbohydrate meals produce more energy and less body fat than the same number of calories from a high-fat meal.

Weigh yourself *only* once every two weeks. Take your vital measurements once every month. Daily fluctuations in water retention and other non-fat-related effects can discourage you. Let the "feel" of your clothes tell you that you are trimmer and leaner.

Building muscle tissue not only burns calories while you exercise, but muscle burns more calories all day long. How chromium helps build muscle tissue is the subject of the next chapter.

REFERENCES

1. *The Easy No-Flab Diet.* Passwater, Richard A. Richard Marek Publishers, NY (1979).
2. *The Slendernow Diet.* Passwater, Richard A. St. Martin's Press, NY (1982).

3. The effects of chromium picolinate supplementation on body composition in different age groups. Kaats, G. R.; Fisher, J. A.; Blum, K. and Adelman, J.A. Abstract represented at the 21st Annual Meeting of the American Aging Association, Denver (October 12, 1991).

4. Effect of chromium picolinate on growth and carcass characteristics of growing-finishing pigs. Page, T.G.; Ward, T.L. and Southern, L.L. *Animal Sci.,* Suppl. 1., 69:356 (1991).

5. Chromium picolinate additions to the diets of growing-finishing pigs. Lindemann, M.D.; Wood, C.M.; Harper, A.F. and Kornegay, E.T. Abstract presented at the Annual Meeting of the American Society of Animal Science (February 1993).

10

Building Strength

In discussing the calorie-restriction approach to aging, I mentioned that I personally did not want to lose too much lean tissue. Chromium picolinate helps build the lean tissue of our vital organs as well as the skeletal muscles that determine our physique.

Biologically active chromium is critically important for muscle growth, because it helps insulin transfer the amino acids through the walls of the muscle cells. Once inside the muscle tissue cells, the amino acids are assembled to repair and make new muscle. Exercise and work requires chromium, and thus they "use up" chromium.[1-4]

Human Studies

We have known that for quite some time, but until studies at Bemidji State University (Minnesota), we did not appreciate just how important chromium picolinate is. At the suggestion of Dr. Gary Evans, Dr. Muriel Gilman and Guy Ott quantified the relationship in two studies of college athletes.

The first study showed that 200 micrograms of chromium as chromium picolinate daily for six weeks resulted in significant muscle growth in athletes compared to those receiving the same training but taking a placebo instead of chromium picolinate.

In this study, ten male students enrolled in a weight training course were randomly assigned into two groups of five men each. All of the students were equally supervised and lifted weights for 40 minutes, twice a week. Neither the athletes nor the instructor knew which subjects were getting the chromium picolinate supplements and which subjects were getting the placebos until the results were compiled.

In the group receiving the chromium picolinate, average total muscle weight (lean body mass) increased a statistically significant 3.5 pounds compared to a gain of less than one-tenth of a pound of muscle in the placebo group.[5] The results were highly statistically significant, that is, not due to chance.

The percentage of weight gain that was muscle was greater in the chromium picolinate group; 73 percent versus 30 percent in the placebo group (4.8 vs. 2.5 pounds).

The tale of the tape was a 1.4 centimeter increase in biceps circumference for the chromium picolinate group versus 1.2 cm for the placebo group. Calf circumference increased a statistically significant 1.15 cm for the chromium picolinate group versus 0.8 cm for the placebo group.

Encouraged by these results, the researchers designed a second study involving 31 football players during the off-season. Again, two groups were randomly assigned and one group received the chromium picolinate and the other a placebo. Again, neither the football players nor the researchers knew who was getting which supplement. All athletes received equal supervision and trained with weights for one hour, four times a week.

When the study was completed, it was found that those who received the chromium picolinate supplements gained an average of 5.7 pounds of muscle tissue, compared to 3.9 pounds in those taking the placebo.[5] Statistically, this 44 percent greater increase is very significant.

A third supporting study was conducted at Louisiana State University. One of the researchers was Deborah Hasten, an award-winning bodybuilder herself, who at that time was a graduate student working toward her doctorate in exercise physiology. This preliminary study was also a placebo-controlled, double-blind study that measured increases in arm, chest and thigh circumferences, with and without 200 micrograms of chromium picolinate daily. However, no measurement of chromium already existing in the diet was performed, nor was the diet controlled in any way.

This study spoke well for the benefit of exercise in increasing lean tissue and decreasing fat. The researchers noted, "all groups gained more lean body mass than body weight, due to a concurrent decrease in body fat." However, the benefit of chromium picolinate was noted. "Both the females and males taking chromium picolinate had significantly greater absolute increases for the sum of the chest, arm, and thigh circumferences than the placebo groups (p = 0.0344). Perhaps the chromium picolinate was responsible for a slight increase in girth at these muscle sites."

The improvement with chromium picolinate averaged 3.4 cm, as opposed to only 1.2 cm without.[6] This study showed a dramatic benefit of chromium picolinate for women, but not for men.

This is not unexpected in science, especially when the number of people studied is small. Most people are aware that the studies used to elucidate the effects of cholesterol, fats, caffeine, saccharine, etc. are sometimes conflicting until several studies with large numbers of people are completed. As the researchers noted, "perhaps the females were consuming diets that were more deficient in chromium than the males. Alternately, a dose-dependent relationship could be in effect. Since the males started out with a significantly greater body weight and lean body weight than the females, they may have benefited from a greater dosage."

A later study at a San Antonio weight-loss clinic also shows that chromium picolinate increases muscle tissue without an increase in exercise. This is the same study discussed in the previous chapter on trimming fat. The volunteers were given chromium picolinate in two nutritional drinks each day for 72 days. They were not placed on diets or told to exercise. On average, the chromium picolinate supplemented group lost 4.2 pounds of fat accompanied by a 1.4 pound increase in muscle tissue. The corresponding results in those not receiving the chromium picolinate were a 0.4 pound fat loss and a 0.2 pound lean tissue gain.[7]

Animal Studies

Animal studies show the same results. The difference here is that the animals did not train or exercise. The chromium picolinate was merely added to their diets, and no changes were made in their routine. Of course, there were no psychological factors involved with the animals.

The animal studies are the same ones discussed in the previous chapter, but here we examine the muscle growth, rather than the fat loss. One study was conducted at Louisiana State University and the other at Virginia Polytechnical Institute.

The Louisiana State University animal study showed that selected lean tissues increased between 7 and 18 percent, with a 21 percent decrease in carcass fat.[8]

The Virginia Polytechnical Institute study reached substantially the similar conclusions: the addition of only 200 parts per billion of chromium as chromium picolinate to the diet of growing pigs increased their pork chop size while reducing back fat.[9]

REFERENCES

1. Effects of aerobic exercise and training on the trace minerals chromium, zinc and copper. Campbell, Wayne and Anderson, Richard A. *Sports Med.* 4:9-18 (1987).

2. Exercise effects on chromium absorption and retention by rats. Polansky, Marilyn M.; Campbell, Wayne and Anderson, Richard A. *Federation Proceed.* 46:1007 (1987).

3. Strenuous exercise may increase dietary needs for chromium and zinc. Anderson, Richard A.; Polansky, Marilyn M.; Bryden, Noella A. and Guttman, Helene N. The 1984 Olympic Scientific Congress Proceedings, V II(1986). *Sport, Health and Nutrition.* Katch, Frank I., Editor.

4. Exercise effects on chromium excretion of trained and untrained men consuming a constant diet. Anderson, Richard A.; Bryden, Noella A.; Polansky Marilyn M. and Dcuster, Patricia A. *J. Appl. Physiol.* 64:249 (1988),

5. The effect of chromium picolinate on insulin controlled parameters in humans. Evans, Gary W. *Internat. J. Biosocial Med. Res.* 11(2); 163-80 (1989).

6. Effects of chromium picolinate on beginning weight training students. Hasten, Deborah L.; Rome, E. P.; Franks, B. D. and Hegsted, M. *Intl. J. Sport Nutrition* 2:343-50 (1992).

7. The effects of chromium picolinate supplementation on body composition in different age groups. Kaats, G. R.; Fisher, J. A. and Blum, K. *Age* 14:138 (1991).

8. Effect of chromium picolinate on growth and carcass characteristics of growing-finishing pigs. Page, T. G.; Ward, T. L. and Southern, L. L. *J. Animal Sci.* 69(Suppl. 1). Abst. #403, presented at the 83rd Annual Meeting Laramie, Wyoming (August 6-9, 1991).

9. Chromium picolinate additions to diets of growing-finishing pigs. Lindemann, M. D.; Wood, C. M.; Harper, A. F. and Kornegay, E. T. Abstract presented at the Annual Meeting of the American Society of Animal Science (February 1993).

11

Most People are Chromium Deficient and Age Prematurely

STUDIES consistently show that most people are deficient in the essential trace mineral chromium.[1] The result is that we age too fast, die too soon, feel tired, gain weight, and develop diseases such as heart disease and diabetes.[2]

Scientists at the United States Department of Agriculture (USDA) have repeatedly warned that most people are not getting adequate amounts of chromium in their diets. The problem has existed for some time due to the increasing reliance on highly processed "refined-food" diets, which are high-sugar and high-fat diets.

Even when whole foods such as fruits and vegetables are eaten, the diet may still be low in chromium. Whereas most minerals that are essential for humans are also essential for plants, chromium, like iodine and selenium, is not essential for plants. Therefore, plants may thrive in chromium-deficient soil. Such plants will contain little chromium.

However, the chromium deficiency problem was not properly recognized until recently, because previous analyses of diets rarely examined chromium levels. In the few studies that did consider chromium content, unreliable analytical procedures and laboratory contamination resulted in falsely high values for chromium.

In 1982, I warned that "unrecognized chromium deficiencies may be one of the most serious nutritional problems today."[2] I based this warning on my gerontological studies showing that body stores of chromium in persons eating refined-food diets decreased dramatically with age, whereas persons eating whole-food diets maintained a normal supply of chromium in their bodies *at all ages*.

Others have noted that the progressive decline in chromium tissue levels with age in U.S. citizens is greater than in many foreign populations.[3] Populations having low heart disease and diabetes have tissue levels 2.5 to 13 times the levels of U. S. citizens at any given age. Most normal diets before the era of modern food processing contained more chromium.

A 1979 study indicated that most contemporary diets were well below 50 micrograms, the lowest level of the recommended range of chromium intake.[4] This study most likely was overgenerous because of the analytical problems. The National Academy of Sciences' recommendation for chromium is 50 to 200 micrograms daily. The low end of this range, 50 micrograms, is far from being an *optimal* amount. This 50 micrograms should be considered the bare minimum.

From 1980 through 1985 three studies from the United States, England, and Finland all found that the typical dietary intake for chromium was 30 micrograms daily, roughly one-half of the lowest amount recommended.[5-7]

In the 1985 USDA study, Drs. Richard Anderson and Adrianne Kozlovsky found that more than 90 percent of diets were below the lowest level of the recommended daily chromium intake. They reported that there were as many diets containing less than one-fifth the lowest recommended level as there were at or above the lowest recommended level.[7] About 60 percent of people received less than half of the lowest recommended level.

In 1992, Dr. Anderson reported on his study of 22 well-balanced diets designed by USDA nutritionists. He found them, too, to be deficient in chromium. The diets averaged only about 13 micrograms of chromium per 1,000 calories.[8]

In that study, Dr. Anderson also reported that chromium supplementation normalized blood sugar levels and lowered cholesterol and triglycerides. After his 1985 study, Dr. Anderson told reporter Franklin Ruehi, "There are no adverse side effects from taking a maximum of 200 micrograms of chromium a day. People are going to have more energy and feel better."

Dr. Norman Kaplan, professor of internal medicine at the University of Texas Southwestern Medical Center at Dallas, added, *"Every adult should take a daily chromium supplement of from 50 to 200 micrograms."* (My italics.)

Professor Matti Tolonen, M.D. of the University of Helsinki is an advisor to the World Health Organization, a member of the scientific boards of the *British Journal of Nutritional Medicine* and *International Clinical Nutrition Review*. Dr. Tolonen recognizes that not all physicians have been exposed to this new information about widespread chromium deficiency. He notes, "Experts are still in disagreement about who needs chromium supplementation...In any case, supplementation is required for the elderly, for diabetics and for people with heart and cardiovascular problems, since these groups are particularly exposed to the risks of chromium deficiency."[9]

People Often Use More Chromium Than They Eat

That's only half of the problem! Not only do people eat diets low in chromium, these diets use up more chromium than they supply. Cereals, grains and sugars in their whole or natural unrefined state are chromium sources. However, food processing removes up to 80 percent of the chromium in these whole foods.[3]

Consumption of high-sugar diets increases chromium excretion by 10 to 300 percent.[10] The body needs this chromium to burn the foods for energy. When chromilum is inadequately supplied, much of the food energy is not burned but is stored in your cells as fat.

REFERENCES

1. Chromium metabolism and its role in disease processes in man. Anderson, Richard A. *Clin. Physiol.* 4:31-41 (1986).

2. *GTF Chromium.* Passwater,Richard A. Keats Publishing, Inc., New Canaan, CT, (1982).

3. Chromium. Pi-Sunyer, F. X. and Offenbacher, E. G. *Nutrition Review's Present Knowledge in Nutrition* (5th ed.). The Nutrition Foundation, Washington, D.C., p 578 (1984).

4. Chromium in Nutrition and Metabolism. Riales, R. Elsevier/North-Holland Biomedical Press, 199-212 (1979).

5. Mineral element content of Finnish foods. Koivistoinen, P. *Acta Agric. Scand.,* Suppl. 22 (1980).

6. The uptake and excretion of chromium by the elderly. Bunker, W.; Lawson, M. D.; Delves, H. T. and Clayton, B. E. *Amer. J. Clin. Nutr.* 39:799-802 (1984).

7. Chromium intake, absorption and excretion of subjects consuming self-selected diets. Anderson, Richard A. and Kozlovsky, A. S. *Amer. J. Clin. Nutr.* 41:1177-83 (1985).

8. *********** Anderson, Richard A. *Biological Trace Element Research* (January-March 1992). (Also see USDA/ARS *Scientific Resarch News,* (November 1991).

9. *Vitamins and Minerals in Health and Nutrition.* Tolonen, M. D., Matti. Simon & Schuster Internat. (Ellis Horwood Ltd.) Chichester, England (1990).

10. Effects of diets high in simple sugars on urinary chromium losses. Kozlovsky, Adrianne S.; Moser, Phylis B.; Reiser, Sheldon and Anderson, Richard A. *Metabolism* 35(6)515-8 (1986).

12

The Remarkable Safety of Chromium Picolinate

THE MANY studies in humans and other animals described throughout this book show that chromium picolinate is indeed effective. Equally important, chromium picolinate is safe. Keep in mind that no university or hospital ethics review committee would ever allow such studies if the product being tested was not clearly shown in advance to be safe. Both acute and chronic toxicity tests of chromium picolinate have established that it is completely nontoxic at nutritional levels. **However, diabetics should have their blood sugar level monitored because of chromium's role as an insulin helper.**

In considering safety, let's look at the chemical parts of the chromium complex, and then the entire complex itself. Chromium picolinate is not a simple molecule. It is a complex called a chelate, in which a chromium ion is protected by three molecules of picolinic acid. Chromium is safe; picolinic acid is safe; and chromium picolinate is safe.

First of all, there are two forms of chromium, but only one form is a nutrient. Nutritional chromium has a valence or oxidation state of "plus three." This has to do with the number of electrons that are readily available to combine with other atoms or electrons. In other words, a molecule of chromium that has lost three electrons, so that it has an electrical charge of +3, is called trivalent chromium.

The chromium in chromium picolinate is trivalent chromium, of course. Trivalent chromium is considered virtually nontoxic, even in amounts many times greater than needed for nutritional purposes.

Recommended Dietary Allowances puts it this way: "The toxicity of trivalent chromium, the chemical form that occurs in diets, is so low that there is a substantial margin of safety between the amounts normally consumed and those considered to have harmful effects. No adverse effects were seen in rats and mice consuming 5 milligrams of chromium per liter of drinking water throughout their lifetimes, and no toxicity was observed in rats exposed to 100 milligrams per kilogram of diet."[1]

In the sixth edition of *Present Knowledge in Nutrition,* it is noted that "the therapeutic-toxic dose ratio for chromium of 1:10,000 means that intakes of trivalent chromium that will produce a physiological effect are quite safe."[2]

In *Toxicants Occurring Naturally in Foods,* the "toxicity" of chromium is listed at "about one milligram per 100 grams of body weight."[3] This would be 700,000 micrograms for a 154-pound person and compares to the 50 to 200 microgram safe and effective range recommended in the RDA.[1] Thus, chromium is the safest of all trace minerals, and ranks with vitamin C and vitamin E in terms of proven safety.

Now, let's look at the picolinate portion of the chromium picolinate complex. Picolinic acid is a natural amino acid derivative. Don't be put off by the "acid" part of the name — amino acids and their derivative acids are very weak acids. While picolinic acid is found in many foods ranging from milk to yeast, keep in mind that our bodies produce picolinic acid in the liver and kidneys from an amino acid. Human milk contains much more picolinic acid than cow's milk. It may be that picolinic acid is used in our bodies to help absorb minerals such as chromium and zinc from our foods. This is discussed in Dr. Gary Evans's Good Health Guide called *The Picolinates.*[4]

It is estimated that we humans produce from 5 to 20 milligrams or more of picolinic acid in our bodies daily. This is far more than the 1.4 milligrams of picolinic acid that accompanies each 200 micrograms of chromium in 1.6

milligrams of chromium picolinate. Under some conditions, picolinic acid itself serves as a beneficial nutrient, and has even shown antitumor activity.[5,6]

At Bemidji State University in Minnesota, Dr. Evans tested the safety of picolinic acid in a standard LD_{50} toxicity test using laboratory rats. He determined the LD_{50} toxicity — the "lethal dose" that would kill 50 percent of the test animals — of *free* picolinic acid to be 750 milligrams of picolinic acid per kilogram of body weight. This is equivalent to 52.5 grams (52,500 milligrams) of picolinic acid for a 154-pound person.

It is important to note that if the picolinic acid were not "free," that is, not attached to minerals such as chromium or zinc, it would be toxic at that level. But, if the picolinic acid were chelated with zinc or chromium, such as in zinc picolinate or chromium picolinate, it would be nontoxic.

Dr. Evans reports, "We could not get enough chromium picolinate into the animals to produce any adverse effects. From our studies, we estimate that the LD_{50} for oral chromium picolinate to be in excess of 2.2 grams per kilogram of body weight, which is equivalent to 156 grams (156,000 milligrams or 156,000,000 micrograms) of chromium picolinate for a 154-pound person. This is a hundred thousand times greater than the nutritional amount (1.6 milligrams) and such an imbalance certainly could not be achieved from taking chromium picolinate supplements.

The difference between free picolinic acid and chelated picolinic acid is that free picolinic acid can pick up and carry away available minerals. Chelated picolinic acid, however, is already saturated with a mineral. If the body separates the chromium from the picolinic acid, the small amount of picolinic acid can be used for tryptophan metabolism, added to the picolinic acid pool to help in the absorption of other minerals, or used to transport or carry away other minerals. The net result of all of these actions is a beneficial gain in mineral nutriture.

How Much Chromium Picolinate Should I Take?

By now, you have read that the safe and effective range for chromium intake is 50 to 200 micrograms per day. You have also learned that many forms of chromium are poorly absorbed, but that chromium picolinate is not only efficiently absorbed, it is also very bioavailable, meaning that it is very well utilized by the body. Chromium picolinate has been proven effective at 200 micrograms of chromium (which is provided by 1.6 milligrams of chromium picolinate). When buying mineral supplements, read the label carefully to ensure that you are getting the amounts that you wish. The label should specify the "elemental" amount of the mineral and the form the mineral is in. The ingredients list should have a column for the minerals which is followed by the form in parenthesis and the amount column should specify "elemental." It should look something like the following:

Mineral	*Amount (elemental)*
chromium (picolinate)	200 mcg

Some manufacturers do not state these important facts in a clear manner. If the list of ingredients does not state the mineral content in terms of its "elemental" content and also specify the mineral form, then check the side panel. In the case of chromium picolinate, the side panel should state something like, "contains 200 micrograms of chromium (elemental) as 1,600 micrograms of chromium picolinate."

You may remember, also, that some of the studies were performed with up to 800 micrograms of chromium daily. I know of other unpublished studies in which up to 2,000 micrograms were taken daily. Just what is the optimal amount to take as a supplement?

Keep in mind that the studies were performed under close medical supervision. We may not know what the optimal intake is, but it is certainly above 200 micrograms per day. However, we do know that 200 micrograms of chromium as 1.6 milligrams of chromium picolinate is *safe and effective*.

Therefore, my advice is to take this proven safe and effective amount as a dietary supplement if you eat a reasonably balanced diet that is low-to-moderate in refined sugars.

If, on the other hand, your diet is not well balanced or is rather high in refined sugars, you might consider starting with 400 micrograms of chromium for a week or two, then dropping to 200 micrograms as a maintenance level.

The need for chromium appears to be related to body size. Big people seem to need more than small people. It's also related to sugar consumption. Soft drinks and candy substantially increase the requirement as shown by several studies. And studies also show that active people need more than sedentary people. So a level of 200 to 400 micrograms daily, based upon these factors would appear prudent for health. Will this also be the ideal range to slow the aging process? Only time will tell.

REFERENCES

1. *Recommended Dietary Allowances* (10th ed.). Food and Nutrition Board, Commission on Life Sciences, National Research Council. National Academy Press, Washington, DC (1989).

2. *Present Knowledge in Nutrition.* Brown, Myrtle L., editor. International Life Sciences Institute, Nutrition Foundation, Washington, DC (1990).

3. *Toxicants Occurring Naturally in Foods.* National Academy Press, Washington, DC (1973).

4. *The Picolinates.* Evans, Gary. Good Health Guide, Keats Publishing, Inc., New Canaan, CT (1989).

5. Effects of dietary picolinate on mice deprived of tryptophan, niacin and vitamin B-6. Van Winkle, Lon J.; Doman, Daniel R. and Campione, Allan L. *J. Nutr. Sci. Vitaminol.* 29:701-7 (1983).

6. Antitumor activity of picolinic acid in CBA/J mice. Leuthauser, Susan W.C.; Oberley, Larry W. and Oberley, Terry. *J. Nat. Can. Inst.* 68(1):123-6 (1982).

FOR FURTHER READING

Major authors and publishers of health and nutrition books endorse the health benefits of chromium picolinate.

The Chromium Program, Jeffrey Fisher, M.D. New York: Harper & Row, Publishers, 1990.

The Doctors' Vitamin and Mineral Encyclopedia, Sheldon Saul Hendler, M.D., Ph.D., New York: Simon & Schuster, 1990.

The Princeton Plan, Edwin Heleniak, M.D., New York: St. Martin's Press, 1990.

The Doctor's Book of Home Remedies, Emmaus, Pa.: Rodale Press, 1990

The Picolinates, Gary W. Evans, Ph.D. New Canaan, Conn.: Keats Publishing, Inc., 1989.

The Purification Prescription, Sheldon Saul Hendler, M.D., Ph.D. New York: William Morrow & Co., Inc., 1991.

The New Supernutrition, Richard A. Passwater, Ph.D. New York: Pocket Books/Simon & Schuster, 1991.

The Best Treatment, Isadore Rosenfield, M.D. New York: Simon & Schuster, 1991.

99 Secrets for a Longer, Healthier Life, Julian M. Whitaker, M.D. Phillips Publishing, Inc., 1991.

How to Lose Wheight Without Dieting, Julian M. Whitaker, M.D. Phillips Publishing, Inc., 1991.

Chromium Picolinate, Richard A. Passwater, Ph.D. New Canaan, Conn.: Keats Publishing,, 1992.

Longevity: The Science off Staying Young, Kathy Keeton, New York: Viking Publishing, 1992.

Dr. Atkins' New Diet Revolution, Robert C. Atkins, M.D. New York: M. Evans & Company, Inc., 1992.